MEAL PREP

Complete Beginner's Guide To Save
Time And Eat Healthier With Batch
Cooking For The Ketogenic Diet

ELIZABETH WELLS

TABLE OF CONTENTS

Free Bonus
The Best Foods To Eat On A Ketogenic Diet

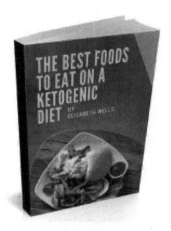

Discover the best foods to eat on a ketogenic diet. You'll learn the different food groups that you should eat to follow the keto diet correctly and start improving your health right now.

Go to **www.eepurl.com/cUqOlH** to download the guide for free.

Introduction

Congratulations on purchasing this book and thank you for doing so.

The following chapters will discuss everything that you need to know to get started with meal prepping. Meal prepping can be good for the whole family, helping you to save money, eat healthy foods, and to save a lot of time. And when you combine it with the ketogenic diet, you are sure to get the weight loss benefits that you are looking for.

Inside this guidebook, you will learn all the basics that you need to know about meal prepping on the ketogenic diet. We will talk about how to meal prep, how to avoid some of the common mistakes that beginners make with meal prepping, and even some of the basics of the ketogenic diet. We will then move on to the best 101 recipes that fit the ketogenic diet and will help you meal prep ahead of time.

When you are ready to lose weight with the ketogenic diet and you want to get started with meal prepping to save time and money, make sure to check out this guidebook!

There are plenty of books on this subject on the market, thanks again for choosing this one! Every effort was made to ensure it is full of as much useful information as possible, please enjoy!

Chapter 1
Understanding the Ketogenic Diet

The ketogenic diet is a low carb diet that is designed to make the body burn fat for energy, rather than glucose. This process, known as ketosis, is able to produce ketones, which is where the ketogenic diet gets its name.

This diet works because it switches out the main source of energy the body uses. Carbs are a favorite food source in the body. It is able to break it down into glucose, which is easy for the body to digest. Without a steady intake of these carbs, the body will either feel lethargic and tired, or it will start to use protein as a form of energy.

However, if you limit your protein a bit (enough to force the body to not use it, but you will still eat enough to keep the muscles strong), the body will start to burn fat as a primary fuel source. This often results in weight loss. You have to make sure that you are limiting your carbs enough that the body won't resort back to burning these as fuel, or the diet won't work.

The biggest indicator about whether the diet is ketogenic is how many carbs it restricts. For the most part, you will need to stay below 50 grams of carbs each day to be considered ketogenic. There are other diet plans that are similar, but they allow for more carbs.

Reaching a state of ketosis is critical when it comes to the ketogenic diet. Ketosis means that the body is not receiving enough glucose to keep it running, so it starts to look for fat to burn as energy. During this process, ketones are created in order to burn up the fat, which is why you are able to check for the level of ketones in your urine to determine if you are in ketosis.

You will find that fat is a much better form of fuel that carbs. When you eat carbs, you are putting your body on a vicious cycle of energy when you take in the carbs, and a big crash when the energy is gone. While you may feel lethargic when the glucose is used, there are still a ton of calories that you have consumed and it is hard to burn them off. The extra glucose in the body will then end up as fat on the body.

But, when it comes to fat as an energy source, things are different. You will be able to burn through the fat quickly, both the fats that you eat on this diet plan and the fat that is built up on your body. You will have a lot of extra energy, eat fewer calories, and lose the weight that you have always wanted.

The most important thing for you to keep track of when you are on this diet plan is the macronutrients. If you stray from these too much, you will kick the body out of ketosis and not get the weight loss that you are looking for.

Of course, you need to consume most of your

calories on this diet plan in fats. These need to be healthy fats like olive oils, fats from dairy products, and fats from animal products. Eating adequate amounts of fats will ensure that you are providing the body with the energy tat it needs to get through the day. The ketogenic diet requires that you eat at least 70 percent of your calories from fat.

Next, you need to take in moderate amounts of protein. It is important to take in enough protein in your diet to ensure that the muscles are healthy and don't start to deteriorate. You should eat about 20 percent of your calories from protein. Eating options like fish and ground beef can provide you with the protein and the fat content that you need.

And finally, you need to limit your carb intake. It is estimated that you take in about 5 percent of your calories from carbs during the day. And when you consume carbs, they should be healthy options like low-carb fruits and vegetables to provide you with the nutrients that you need.

Following the ketogenic diet does require some planning ahead to see results, but it is one of the best ones to help you to lose weight. And with the help of the recipes in this guidebook and the meal prep basics that follow, you will be able to see how delicious and easy this diet plan can be.

Chapter 2
The Basics of Meal Planning

Meal planning or prepping is the best process that you can use to ensure that you are able to build healthy and delicious meals each day. You don't have to worry about making decisions at the last minute or that you are not going to be able to keep away from temptations when you are hungry. You know what you are going to eat each day, and you have the ingredients for it all ready, ahead of time. There are a lot of benefits that come with meal planning including:

- Saving money: Meal planning allows you to buy things in bulk, look for ads and specials, and to split up the meals so that you can save your money.
- Saving time: You will have to spend a lot of time one day preparing the meals, but you can work on a few meals at once, saving yourself a lot of time compared to nightly cooking.
- Controlling portions: It is much easier to make the meals last here because you are able to divide up the food and make the right portions for your needs.
- Good meals even when you are busy: Even if

you have a busy night, meal planning will help you out since the meals are ready for you ahead of time.

- Eating healthier: Since the meals are ready ahead of time, you can choose how healthy you would like them to be. You will also be less likely to give in to your cravings when the meal is already planned for you.

Principles of meal prep

The major reason that a lot of people choose to go with meal planning to help them out is to eat healthier. While it is true that it makes life easier and it helps you to save money, a lot of people are worried about following a certain diet plan so they decide to get started with meal planning.

Before you are able to get started with this great process, you need to understand some of the main principles that come with meal planning, such as:

- Simple meals first: When you first get started, you need to start out slow. Pick out meals that are easy to put together. Pick five to ten recipes that don't take you long to make but are your favorites and keep those around. As you get more used to meal planning, you can add in more variety later.
- Batch cook: This means that you will double, or even triple, the recipe. This saves time, allows you to purchase in bulk, and makes things easier.
- Creative reuse: Think of ways that you are able to reuse the leftovers of a meal. If you make a chicken meal one day, for example, can you shred it up and use it as a sandwich the

next day? This helps you to avoid waste without making things boring.

- Add the vegetables and salads: These are simple to use and can fit well into most diet plans. Cook some up ahead of time so they are always ready.
- Pick out recipes with ingredients you already have: You don't need to make meal prepping complicated. Pick recipes that have ingredients you are familiar with and may already have in your home; you are more likely to eat these.

Meal prepping can really make a big difference in your life. It will help you to lose weight, save money, save time, and just makes life easier than ever.

Chapter 3
The Common Mistakes Made by Meal Prepping Beginners

As a beginner in meal planning, you want to make sure that you are using your time wisely. You don't want to waste ingredients, waste time, or do other things that take away from the benefits that come with this kind of prep. Some of the common mistakes that you need to avoid as a beginner include:

Not building a balanced meal

Eating too much of one food, and not enough of another, can mess up the day. The recipes below will help you to get the right balance between the carbs, protein, and fats that you need on the ketogenic diet. But if you are choosing from other sources, make sure that you are balancing out the meals so that your macronutrients are still in place.

Preparing it all in one day

It may be tempting to prepare all the food in one day, but have you ever tasted chicken, or other meat, after it has been in the fridge for a week?

These often taste poorly and you will not want to eat it. You can choose a few options. Some people just make meals for a few days at a time and call that good. If you need to make a lot of meals at once, consider freezing them to keep everything fresh for when you need it.

Never mixing it up

Eating the exact same things, or things that are similar, can get boring. It is important to think about the meals that you are preparing and that you pick out a variety of meals that will taste good. Eating chicken every day for a month is going to get boring, but mixing up the meals to include some fish, some beef, some turkey, and even some vegetarian options can make things easier.

There are a lot of great recipes out there, and many of them are simple and easy to follow. Just find some of your favorite ketogenic friendly recipes and add them into the mix, and it will be easy to stay interested in your meal plan for a long time to come.

Not stocking up the kitchen

It is impossible to cook up these healthy meals without planning ahead a bit. If you are working on a recipe and you don't have the ingredients, you may reach for a substitute that is not that healthy. For example, you may need brown rice in a recipe and instead use white pasta when you are out. Always plan ahead and know what you need for all of your recipes to make things easier.

Not storing properly

The containers that you store the meals in can

actually affect how much food you are going to make and eat. If you are picking out containers that are huge, your portion sizes are going to be really large as well. Pick out portion-controlled containers, or ones that are only as big as the amount of food that your family will eat. You may find that some of the meals can be divided in two, saving you even more money.

You should also consider whether the containers are going to seal up tight as well. Otherwise, the meals are going to be rubbery and tasteless. Luckily, there are a lot of different options that you can choose one so pick the one that works the best for your lifestyle.

Picking out complicated cooking methods

You do not need to pick out meals that are going to take hours to put together and need the most complicated cooking method possible. It is fine to keep things simple, especially when it comes to your meal planning. For example, there is nothing wrong with doing a few recipes each time that use the slow cooker. You simply need to throw the ingredients in the slow cooker and the meal is done. You can always mix it up with different cooking methods but making it simple is the name of the game with meal planning.

Meal planning can be one of the best ways to save you a lot of money and time. But there are some mistakes that can take away from all the benefits that you can get with meal planning. Make sure to avoid these common mistakes and you will be a meal planning professional in no time.

Chapter 4
Easy Breakfast Meals to Start the Day

Sausage and Egg Keto Sandwich

Prep time: 5 minutes
Cooking time: 10 minutes
Servings: 1 (multiply by how many days you want to eat this)

What's in it

- Avocado slices
- Cheddar cheese (2)
- Sausage patties (2)
- Mayo (1 Tbsp.)
- Butter (1 Tbsp.)
- Eggs (2)

How's it done

1. Take out a pan and heat the butter up. Add some molds into the pan and break the eggs inside, mixing with a fork.
2. Cook the eggs for 3 minutes before taking out of the heat. Take one of the eggs and add half the cheese, one cooked sausage patty, and half the mayo.
3. Place the other sausage on top of the avocado and finish with the cheese. Put the rest of the mayo on the egg and complete your sandwich.

Nutrition
Calories: 880
Fats: 82g
Carbs: 10.5g
Protein: 32g

Keto Cereal

Prep time: 5 minutes
Cooking time: 0 minutes
Servings: 3

What's in it

- Milk
- Toasted flax seeds (1 c.)
- Toasted macadamia pieces (1 c.)
- Toasted walnut pieces (1 c.)
- Cinnamon (.5 tsp.)
- Salt
- Sweetener of choice
- Shredded coconut (1.5 c.)

How's it done

1. To make this dish, combine together all of the ingredients. Heat up if you would like and serve with the almond milk.

Nutrition
Calories: 350
Fats: 24g.
Carbs: 2 g
Protein: 22g

Ham and Cheese Waffles

Prep time: 10 minutes
Cooking time: 4 minutes per waffle.
Servings: 2

What's in it

- Eggs (8)
- Baking powder (1 tsp.)
- Basil and paprika
- Grated cheddar cheese (2 oz.)
- Chopped ham steak (2 oz.)
- Salt (1 tsp.)
- Melted butter (12 Tbsp.)

How's it done

2. Separate four of the eggs into a bowl and set the other four to the side. Add the salt, butter, baking powder, and powder to the egg yolks and whisk together.
3. Slowly fold in the ham. Whisk the egg whites with the salt until they are stiff.
4. Now fold half of the whites into the egg yolk mixture. Let it set for a few minutes before folding in the rest of the egg white.
5. Add a bit of this to the waffle maker and cook for four minutes until done. Repeat with the rest of the batter.

Nutrition
Calories: 620
Fats: 50g
Carbs: 1g
Protein: 45g

Baked Eggs with Avocado

Prep time: 10 minutes
Cooking time: 15 minutes
Servings: 4

What's in it

- Eggs (4)
- Sliced avocado (2)
- Garlic powder (1 pinch)
- Salt (1 pinch)
- Pepper (1 pinch)
- Grated Parmesan cheese (1 handful)

How's it done

1. Allow the oven to 350. Cut up the avocado and scoop out a quarter of the flesh. Add them to a muffin tin.
2. Sprinkle on the seasonings to the avocado. Crack an egg into each half and sprinkle on the cheese.
3. Place this into the oven. After 15 minutes, you can take them out and enjoy.

Nutrition
Calories: 261
Fats: 20g
Carbs: 3g
Protein: 14g

Bacon Cups

Prep time: 10 minutes
Cooking time: 15 minutes
Servings: 6

What's in it

- Pepper
- Salt
- Cheese (.25 c.)
- Spinach (1 handful)
- Eggs (6)
- Bacon strips (6)

How's it done

1. Heat up the oven to 400 degrees. Fry up the bacon and then drain off the fat.
2. Take out a muffin tin and line with the bacon slices. Press down but allow the ends to stick up.
3. Beat your eggs in a bowl and then drain the spinach off. Chop this up roughly and then add to the eggs.
4. Put a bit of this egg mixture into the muffin tin and sprinkle with the seasonings. Place into the oven.
5. After 15 minutes, the eggs will be done and you can serve.

Nutrition
Calories: 101
Fats: 7g
Carbs: 1g
Protein: 8g

Yogurt Parfait

Prep time: 10 minutes
Cooking time: 0 minutes
Servings: 4

What's in it

- Toasted walnut pieces (1 c.)
- Sweetener
- Shredded coconut (1 c.)
- Full fat yogurt (2 c.)
- Blueberries (4 handfuls)
- Strawberries (4 handfuls)
- Sliced bananas (4)
- Toasted flax seeds (1 c.)
- Macadamia pieces (1 c.)

How's it done

1. Take out a glass serving jar and add three tablespoons of yogurt to the bottom.
2. Add the sweetener, and then a layer of nuts, coconut, and banana. Keep alternating until all ingredients are gone.
3. Pour the rest of the yogurt on top.

Nutrition
Calories: 230
Fats: 15g
Carbs: 9g
Protein: 20g

Cheddar Pancakes

Prep time: 15 minutes
Cooking time: 10 minutes
Servings: 4

What's in it

- Baking powder (1 tsp.)
- Chopped green onion (1 Tbsp.)
- Olive oil (4 Tbsp.)
- Almond meal (2 c.)
- Cheddar cheese (4 oz.)
- Egg whites (4)

How's it done

1. Combine the garlic, onion, cheese, water, and almond meal together and set aside.
2. Whisk the eggs and then add in the baking powder. When these are combined, add in the almond meal mix. Beat until smooth.
3. Heat up some olive oil and swirl to coat. When it is hot, ladle some of the batter onto the skillet and cook for a few minutes.
4. Repeat with the rest of the batter and enjoy.

Nutrition
Calories: 257
Fats: 24g
Carbs: 2g
Protein: 11g

Sausage Breakfast Burgers

Prep time: 25 minutes
Cooking time: 20 minutes
Servings: 4

What's in it

- Olive oil (4 Tbsp.)
- Breakfast sausage (.25 c.)
- American cheese (4 slices)
- Portobello mushroom caps (8)

How's it done

1. Rinse off the mushrooms and dry off. Take out a skillet and heat it up with some olive oil.
2. Add two of the mushroom caps and let them cook for five minutes on each side. Repeat with the rest of the caps.
3. Divide up the sausage into four patties. Wipe off the skillet and reheat it. Add some more oil and then two of the patties. Cook for a few minutes on each side to cook through.
4. Add some cheese on the patties and cook a bit longer. Slice these up and add to the mushroom caps.
5. Repeat with the rest of the ingredients.

Nutrition
Calories: 504
Fats: 41g
Carbs: 10g
Protein: 24g

Blueberry Scones

Prep time: 10 minutes
Cooking time: 15 minutes
Servings: 12

What's in it

- Baking powder (2 tsp.)
- Vanilla (2 tsp.)
- Stevia (.5 c.)
- Raspberries (.75 c.)
- Almond flour (1.5 c.)
- Beaten eggs (3)

How's it done

1. Allow the oven to heat up to 375 degrees and add some parchment paper to a baking sheet.
2. Take out a bowl and beat together the almond flour, eggs, baking powder, vanilla, and stevia. Fold the raspberries in.
3. Scoop this batter onto the baking sheet. Add to the oven. After 15 minutes, take the scones out and let them cool down before serving.

Nutrition
Calories: 133
Fats: 8g
Carbs: 4g
Protein: 2g

Cinnamon Porridge

Prep time: 5 minutes
Cooking time: 5 minutes
Servings: 4

What's in it

- Cinnamon (1 tsp.)
- Stevia (1.5 tsp.)
- Butter (1 Tbsp.)
- Flaxseed meal (2 Tbsp.)
- Oat bran (2 Tbsp.)
- Shredded coconut (.5 c.)
- Heavy cream (1 c.)
- Water (2 c.)

How's it done

1. Combine all of your ingredients into a pot and mix around.
2. Place it on a low flame and bring to a boil. Stir it well when it is boiling and then remove from the heat.
3. Divide into four servings and set aside for a bit to thicken.

Nutrition
Calories: 171
Fats: 16g
Carbs: 6g
Protein: 2g

Scotch Eggs

Prep time: 15 minutes
Cooking time: 25 minutes
Servings: 6

What's in it

- Pepper (.5 tsp.)
- Salt (.33 tp.)
- Garlic powder (1.5 tsp.)
- Breakfast sausage (1.5 c.)
- Peeled hard-boiled eggs

How's it done

1. Allow the oven to heat up to 400 degrees. Add the sausage to a bowl and add the garlic, pepper, and salt.
2. Divide this into 6 equal parts and add to some baking paper. Flatten them out and then place the hard boiled eggs on top. Wrap the sausage around the egg.
3. Arrange onto a baking sheet and place into the oven. After 25 minutes, take these out and allow to cool down.

Nutrition
Calories: 258
Fats: 21g
Carbs: 1g
Protein: 17g

Breakfast Tacos

Prep time: 10 minutes
Cooking time: 5 minutes
Servings: 2

What's in it

- Pepper
- Salt
- Tabasco sauce
- Cilantro sprigs (4)
- Butter (1 Tbsp.)
- Sliced avocado (.5)
- Eggs (4)
- Low carb tortillas (2)

How's it done

1. Whisk the eggs until they are smooth. Take out a skillet and heat up the butter on it.
2. Add the prepared eggs and spread it out. cook until done and then move to a bowl. Warm up the tortillas and then put on a platter.
3. Spread mayo over one side of the tortillas. Divide up the egg on the tortilla and top with the avocado and cilantro. Add the pepper, salt, and pepper sauce.
4. Roll up the tortillas and then serve or store.

Nutrition
Calories: 289
Fats: 27g
Carbs: 6g
Protein: 7g

Vanilla Smoothie

Prep time: 2 minutes
Cooking time: 0
Servings: 1

What's in it

- Whipped cream
- Liquid stevia (3 drops)
- Vanilla (.5 tsp.)
- Ice cubes (4)
- Water (.25 c.)
- Mascarpone cheese (.5 c.)
- Egg yolks (2)

How's it done

1. Take out your blender and add in all the ingredients.
2. Place the lid on top and blend. When the ingredients are well mixed, pour into a glass and serve.

Nutrition
Calories: 650
Fats: 64g
Carbs: 4g
Protein: 12g

Blackberry Egg Bake

Prep time: 10 minutes
Cooking time: 15 minutes
Servings: 4

What's in it

- Chopped rosemary (1 tsp.)
- Orange zest (.5 tsp.)
- Salt
- Vanilla (.25 tsp.)
- Grated ginger (1 tsp.)
- Coconut flour (3 Tbsp.)
- Butter (1 Tbsp.)
- Egg (5)
- Blackberries (.5 c.)

How's it done

1. Allow the oven to heat up to 350 degrees. Take out a blender and add all the ingredients inside to blend well.
2. Pour this into each muffin cup and then add the blackberries on top. Place into the oven to bake.
3. After 15 minutes, take the dish out and store!

Nutrition
Calories: 144
Fats: 10g
Carbs: 2g
Protein: 8.5g

Coconut Pancakes

Prep time: 10 minutes
Cooking time: 5 minutes
Servings: 2

What's in it

- Maple syrup (4 Tbsp.)
- Shredded coconut (.25 c.)
- Salt
- Erythritol (.5 Tbsp.)
- Cinnamon (1 tsp.)
- Almond flour (1 Tbsp.)
- Cream cheese (2 oz.)
- Eggs (2)

How's it done

1. Beat the eggs together before adding in the almond flour and cream cheese.
2. Now add in the rest of the ingredients and stir until well combined.
3. Take out a frying pan and fry the pancakes on both sides. Add to a plate and sprinkle some coconut on top.

Nutrition
Calories: 575
Fats: 51g
Carbs: 3.5g
Protein: 19g

Chocolate Chip Waffles

Prep time: 8 minutes
Cooking time: 10 minutes
Servings: 2

What's in it

- Maple syrup (.5 c.)
- Cacao nibs (50g)
- Salt
- Butter (2 Tbsp.)
- Separated eggs (2)
- Protein powder (2 scoops)

How's it done

1. Take out a bowl and beat the egg whites until soft peaks form. In a second bowl mix the butter, protein powder, and egg yolks.
2. Now fold the egg whites into this mixture and add the cacao nibs and salt.
3. Pour the mixture into a waffle maker and let it cook until golden brown on both sides. Serve with maple syrup.

Nutrition
Calories: 400
Fats: 26g
Carbs: 4.5g
Protein: 34g

Chocolate and Peanut Butter Muffins

Prep time: 20 minutes
Cooking time: 20 minutes
Servings: 6

What's in it

- Eggs (2)
- Almond milk (.33 c.)
- Peanut butter (.33 c.)
- Salt
- Baking powder (1 tsp.)
- Erythritol (.5 c.)
- Almond flour (1 c.)

How's it done

1. Bring out a bowl and mix the salt, baking powder, erythritol, and almond flour together. Add the eggs, almond milk, and peanut butter next.
2. Finally, mix in the cacao nibs before pouring this into a muffin tin.
3. Allow the oven to heat up to 350 degrees. Place the muffin tray into the oven to bake.
4. After 25 minutes, the muffins are done and you can store.

Nutrition
Calories: 265
Fats: 20.5g
Carbs: 2g
Protein: 7.5g

Blender pancakes

Prep Time: 5 minutes:
Cooking time: 5 minutes
Servings: 1

What's in it

- Salt
- Cinnamon
- Protein powder (1 scoop)
- Eggs (2)
- Cream cheese (2 oz.)

How's it done

1. Add the salt, cinnamon, protein powder, eggs, and cream cheese to a blender and combine well.
2. Take out a skillet and fry the batter on both sides until done. Serve warm.

Nutrition
Calories: 450
Fat: 29g
Carbs: 4g
Protein: 41g

Butter Coffee

Prep time: 5 minutes
Cooking time
Servings: 1

What's in it

- Coconut oil (1 Tbsp.)
- Butter (1 Tbsp.)
- Coffee (2 Tbsp.)
- Water (1 c.)

How's it done

1. Bring out a pan and boil the water inside. When the water is boiling, add in the coffee, coconut oil, and butter.
2. Once these are all melted and hot, pour into a cup through a strainer and enjoy.

Nutrition
Calories: 230
Fat: 25g
Carbs: 0g
Protein: 0g

Mocha Chia Pudding

Prep time: 5 minutes
Cooking time: 10 minutes
Servings: 2

What's in it

- Cacao nibs (2 Tbsp.)
- Swerve (1 Tbsp.)
- Vanilla (1 Tbsp.)
- Coconut cream (.33 g)
- Chia seeds (55g)
- Water (2 c.)
- Herbal coffee (2 Tbsp.)

How's it done

1. Brew the herbal coffee with some hot water until the liquid is reduced in half. Strain the coffee before mixing in with the vanilla, swerve, and coconut cream.
2. Add in the chia seeds and cacao nibs net. Pour into some cups and place in the fridge for 30 minutes before serving.

Nutrition
Calories: 257
Fat: 20.25g
Carbs: 2.25g
Protein: 7g

Keto Green Eggs

Prep time: 5 minutes
Cooking time: 12 minutes
Servings:2

What's in it

- Ground cayenne (.25 tsp.)
- Ground cumin (.25 tsp.)
- Eggs (4)
- Chopped parsley (.5 c.)
- Chopped cilantro (.5 c.)
- Thyme leaves (1 tsp.)
- Garlic cloves (2)
- Coconut oil (1 Tbsp.)
- Butter (2 Tbsp.)

How's it done

1. Melt the butter and coconut oil in a skillet before adding the garlic and frying. Add in the thyme, parsley and cilantro and cook another 3 minutes.
2. At this time, add in the eggs and season. Cover with a lid and let this cook for another 5 minutes before serving.

Nutrition
Calories: 311
Fat: 27.5g
Carbs: 4g
Protein: 12.8g

Cheddar Souffles

Prep time: 15 minutes
Cooking time: 25 minutes
Servings: 8

What's in it

- Cheddar cheese (2 c.)
- Heavy cream (.75 c.)
- Cayenne pepper (.25 tsp.)
- Xanthan gum (.5 tsp.)
- Pepper (.5 tsp.)
- Ground mustard (1 tsp.)
- Salt (1 tsp.)
- Almond flour (.5 c.)
- Salt (1 pinch)
- Cream of tartar (.25 tsp.)
- Eggs (6)
- Chopped chives (.25 c.)

How's it done

1. Allow the oven to heat up to 350 degrees. Take out a bowl and mix all the ingredients besides the eggs and cream of tartar together.
2. Separate the egg whites and yolks and add the yolks in with the first mixture. Beat the egg whites and cream of tartar until you get stiff peaks to form.
3. Take this mixture and add into the other mixture. When done, pour into the ramekins and place in the oven.
4. After 25 minutes, these are done and you can serve or store.

Nutrition
Calories: 288   Fat: 21g

Carbs: 3g   Protein: 14g

Ricotta Pie

Prep time: 10 minutes
Cooking time: 30 minutes
Servings: 6

What's in it

- Mozzarella (1 c.)
- Eggs (3)
- Ricotta cheese (2 c.)
- Swiss chard (8 c.)
- Garlic clove (1)
- Chopped onion (.5 c.)
- Olive oil (1 Tbsp.)
- Mild sausage (1 lb.)
- Pepper
- Salt
- Nutmeg
- Parmesan (.25 c.)

How's it done

1. Heat up the garlic, onion, and oil on a pan. When those are warm, add in the swiss chard and fry to make the leaves wilt.
2. Add in the nutmeg and set it aside. In a new bowl, beat the eggs before adding in the cheeses. Now add in the prepared swiss chard mixture.
3. Roll out the sausage and press it into a pie tart. Pour the filing inside. Allow the oven to heat to 350 degrees.
4. Place the pie inside and let it bake. After 30 minutes, it is done and you can store or serve.

Nutrition

Calories: 344   Fat: 27g
Carbs: 4g   Protein: 23g

Chapter 5
Lunch Meals the Caveman Way

Buffalo Chicken Wraps

Prep time: 5 minutes
Cooking time: 10 minutes
Servings: 4

What's in it

- Sliced scallions (2)
- Chicken thighs, chopped (2 lbs.)
- Celery stalks (4)
- Diced green pepper (.5)
- Diced red pepper (.5)
- Lettuce leaves (8)
- Butter (2 Tbsp.)
- Garlic powder (1 tsp.)
- Onion powder (2 tsp.)
- Crumbled blue cheese (.5 c.)

How's it done

1. Melt the butter in a pan and add the celery and peppers. After five minutes, add in the garlic, onion, and chicken. Cook the chicken through.
2. Take the pan off the heat and add the scallions and the cheese.
3. Lay out the lettuce leaves and add a few tablespoons of the mixture on top. Roll up and serve.

Nutrition
Calories: 547   Fats: 37g

Carbs: 3g   Protein: 50g

Prosciutto and Brie Sandwich

Prep time: 5 minutes
Cooking time: 8 minutes
Servings: 2

What's in it

- Pepper
- Salt
- Sesame seeds (1 pinch)
- Butter (2 tsp.)
- Raw spinach (2 c.)
- Mushrooms (6)
- Prosciutto slices (8)
- Brie (4 slices)
- Avocado (1)

How's it done

1. Cook the spinach on the stove for five minutes to wilt. Drain out the extra water.
2. Slice the mushrooms and cook in a pan with the butter. Add in the salt and pepper.
3. Slice the avocado in half. Remove the stone and then slice a bit off the bottom so it stands up.
4. Fill the avocado up with the rest of the ingredients and serve as an open-faced sandwich.

Nutrition
Calories: 482
Fats: 40g
Carbs: 12g
Protein: 16g

ELIZABETH WELLS

Keto Cubano

Prep time: 5 minutes
Cooking time: 0 minutes
Servings: 4

What's in it

- Bib lettuce
- Dijon mustard (2 Tbsp.)
- Mayo (2 Tbsp.)
- Melted butter (1 Tbsp.)
- Sliced Swiss cheese (.25 lb.)
- Cooked pork tenderloin (.33 lb.)
- Sliced cooked ham (.33 lb.)
- Sliced dill pickles

How's it done

1. Mix together the mustard and the mayo and spread over the lettuce.
2. Divide up the meats, cheese, and pickle between the sandwiches and roll them up tightly.
3. Serve right away.

Nutrition
Calories: 472
Fats 36g
Carbs: 7g
Protein: 28g

Keto Monkey Bread

Prep time: 10 minutes
Cooking time: 20 minutes
Servings: 3

What's in it

- Crushed garlic clove (1)
- Basil (1 Tbsp.)
- Melted butter (2 Tbsp.)
- Shredded mozzarella cheese (.75 c.)
- Cubed eggplants (2)

How's it done

1. Allow the oven to heat up to 375 degrees. Prepare a muffin tin.
2. Take out a bowl and combine half the basil, the butter, and the garlic. Place a few pieces of the eggplant into the bottom of each muffin tray.
3. Sprinkle the cheese over it all and drizzle the butter mixture on top of the eggplants.
4. Add to the oven and let it bake until the cheese is browned. After 20 minutes, take out of the oven and store.

Nutrition
Calories: 195
Fats: 15g
Carbs: 6g
Protein: 8g

Roast Beef Cups

Prep time: 3 minutes
Cooking time: 2 minutes
Servings: 1

What's in it

- Cheddar cheese (.5 c.)
- Hot chilis (1.5 Tbsp.)
- Sour cream (1 Tbsp.)
- Roast beef (5 slices, thin)

How's it done

1. Break the beef into smaller parts and then lay in the bottom of a dish, mug or cup. Cover with the sour cream.
2. Add a third of your chili and a third of the cheese. Repeat these steps until the ingredients are used up.
3. Place in the microwave for a few minutes to melt and then serve.

Nutrition
Calories: 270
Fats: 18g
Carbs: 4g
Protein: 23g

Pork Salad

Prep time: 15 minutes
Cooking time: 30 minutes
Servings: 2

What's in it

- Sliced pear (.25)
- Blue cheese (.33 c.)
- Pork belly slices (.5 lb.)
- Olive oil (2 tsp.)
- White wine vinegar (2 Tbsp.)
- Mustard (.5 tsp.)
- Water (1 tsp.)
- Stevia (1 Tbsp.)
- Chopped walnuts (.3 c.)
- Sat (2 tsp.)
- Salad leaves (2 c.)

How's it done

1. Cover the pork with half your oil and then cook it in the oven for 30 minutes.
2. Warm up a pan and add the stevia and water. When the stevia dissolves, add the walnuts and cook for about five minutes.
3. Take the nuts and allow them to cool. While those are cooling, chop the cheese and pear into smaller bits.
4. To make the dressing, add the oil, vinegar, and mustard to a bowl.
5. Take the pork out of the oven and slice into smaller bits. Toss the salad with the dressing before adding the rest of the ingredients and serving.

Nutrition

Calories: 1050   Fats: 55g

Carbs: 5g   Protein: 13g
Baked Chicken Nuggets

Prep time: 20 minutes
Cooking time: 45 minutes
Servings: 4 nuggets

What's in it

- Dried oregano (.5 tsp.)
- Salt (1 tsp.)
- Parmesan cheese (.5 c.)
- Milk (.5 c.)
- Marinara sauce (1 c.)
- Almond flour (1 c.)
- Mozzarella cheese (3 oz.)
- Minced chicken breast (1 lb.)

How's it done

1. Allow the oven to heat up to 350 degrees. Coat a baking dish and set to the side.
2. Combine half the almond flour with the pepper, salt, cheese, and milk in a bowl. Add in the chicken and mix to combine.
3. Divide this into 24 balls and then dredge through the reserved almond flour.
4. Place onto the baking dish and place into the oven. Bake for a total of 20 minutes but flip around halfway through.
5. Once these are done, pour the sauce on top and then dot with some cheese. Place back in the oven.
6. After 15 minutes, take this out of the oven and serve.

Nutrition
Calories: 282   Fats: 12g

Carbs: 11g   Protein: 33g

Grilled Shrimp and Avocado Salad

Prep time: 20 minutes
Cooking time: 5 minutes
Servings: 6

What's in it

- Pepper
- Salt (1 tsp.)
- Garlic powder (1 tsp.)
- Lime juice 2 tsp.)
- Olive oil (4 Tbsp.)
- Chopped onion (.5 c.)
- Bell pepper, chopped (.5 c.)
- Chopped tomato (.5 c.)
- Peeled shrimp (2 lb.)
- Cubed avocados (2)

How's it done

1. Place a grill over a medium heat and let it warm up. While that heats up. Combine the oil, salt, pepper, and garlic powder.
2. Add the shrimp inside and toss to coat. Set aside.
3. Take out another bowl and combine the rest of the ingredients and then place in the fridge until ready to serve.
4. Cook the shrimp for three minutes on each side to cook through. Divide up with the salad.

Nutrition
Calories: 409
Fats: 25g
Carbs: 11g
Protein: 36g

Mediterranean Tuna

Prep time 15 minutes
Cooking time: 0 minutes
Servings: 6

What's in it

- Pepper
- Salt
- Red pepper flakes
- Drained capers (1.5 Tbsp.)
- Lemon juice (1.5 Tbsp.)
- Parsley (.33 c.)
- Quartered green olives (.33 c.)
- Roasted red peppers (.75 c.)
- Olive oil (.75 c.)
- Crumbled feta cheese (1.5 c.)
- Tuna (15 oz.)
- Endives (300 grams)

How's it done

1. Add the tuna into a bowl and crumble it around. Fold in the rest of the ingredients, making sure to mix well.
2. Divide this salad into the six servings and then place into airtight containers to eat when ready.

Nutrition
Calories: 352
Fats: 26g
Carbs: 5g
Protein: 25g

Mac and Cheese

Prep time: 10 minutes
Cooking time: 30 minutes
Servings: 4

What's in it

- Pepper
- Garlic (.25 tsp.)
- Cubed cream cheese (.25 c.)
- Parmesan cheese (.25 c.)
- Mozzarella cheese (.25 c.)
- Cheddar cheese (.5 c.)
- Heavy cream (.5 c.)
- Chopped cauliflower head (1)

How's it done

1. Allow the oven to heat up to 400 degrees. Take out a pot of water and bring it to a boil. Add the cauliflower and boil for a few minutes. Drain it out.
2. Add a skillet to the stove and add the cream. Bring this to a simmer and add the cream cheese. Stir in the mozzarella, cheddar, and garlic and stir around.
3. Turn off the heat and mix the cauliflower. Stir until coated.
4. Prepare a baking dish and add the cauliflower mixture. Sprinkle the Parmesan on top and then place in the oven.
5. After 15 minutes, take out of the oven and cool down.

Nutrition
Calories: 198   Fats: 17g
Carbs: 3g   Protein: 10g

Pork Tenderloin

Prep time: 15 minutes
Cooking time: 20 minutes
Servings: 2

What's in it

- Thyme sprigs (3)
- Rosemary sprigs (3)
- Soy sauce (.75 tsp.)
- Olive oil (1.5 Tbsp.)
- Balsamic vinegar (2 Tbsp.)
- Butter (3 Tbsp.)
- Minced shallot (1)
- Peeled garlic clove (1)
- Pork tenderloin (.75 lb.)

How's it done

1. Allow the oven time to heat up to 475 degrees. Season the pork with pepper and salt.
2. Take out a skillet and then add in the butter and olive oil. Cook the shallot and garlic for a few minutes before adding in the pork.
3. Stir in the rest of the ingredients until they are warm. Add to a baking dish and place in the oven.
4. Cook for about 5 minutes, or until the pork is cooked through. Allow the meat time to cool down before serving.

Nutrition
Calories: 508
Fats: 34g
Carbs: 4g
Protein: 45g

Parmesan Chicken Fingers

Prep time: 15 minutes
Cooking time: 30 minutes
Servings: 6

What's in it

- Pepper
- Salt
- Chili pepper flakes (1 tsp.)
- Chopped thyme (2 Tbsp.)
- Parmesan cheese (1 c.)
- Butter (4 oz.)
- Chopped garlic cloves (4)
- Chicken breast (2 lbs.)

How's it done

1. Allow the oven to heat up to 350 degrees. Place a pan on the stove and add the butter to melt.
2. Stir the garlic in and then set aside for a bit. Take out a bowl and combine the pepper, salt, chili pepper, parmesan cheese, and thyme.
3. Rinse out the chicken and then slice into 24 fingers. Coat first in the garlic butter mixture and then into the cheesy mixture. Place in a baking sheet and into the oven.
4. After 30 minutes, the chicken fingers are done. Allow them to cool.

Nutrition
Calories: 370
Fats: 20g
Carbs: 6g
Protein: 40g

Ham and Green Bean Salad

Prep time: 15 minutes
Cooking time: 0 minutes
Servings: 4 persons

What's in it

- Red wine vinegar (1.5 Tbsp.)
- Olive oil (2 Tbsp.)
- Parsley (2.5 Tbsp.)
- Chopped hard boiled eggs (1)
- Chopped Spanish ham (1 oz.)
- Diced red bell pepper (1)
- White onion, minced (1)
- Steamed green beans (.5 lb.)

How's it done

1. Rinse and drain the green beans. Combine together the pepper, salt, vinegar, and olive oil and mix well.
2. Divide up the green beans and then add the parsley, egg, peppers, ham, and onion. Add the dressing.
3. Cover and save for two days.

Nutrition
Calories: 102
Fats: 8g
Carbs: 5g
Protein: 4g

Cheesy Avocado Patties

Prep time: 15 minutes
Cooking time: 10 minutes
Servings: 2

What's in it

- Pepper
- Salt
- Cheddar cheese (2 slices)
- Peeled avocado (1)
- Ground beef (.5 lb.)

How's it done

1. Preheat the grill or broiler. Divide the beef into two patties and season with the pepper and salt.
2. Grill or broil the beef patties until they are cooked through.
3. Move to a platter and add the cheese on top. To store, wrap in some foil and leave in the fridge.

Nutrition
Calories: 568
Fats: 43g
Carbs: 9g
Protein:38g

Feta Cheese Salad

Prep time: 10 minutes
Cooking time: 20 minutes
Servings: 8

What's in it

- Chopped spring onions (2)
- Roasted pistachios (50g)
- Feta cheese (150g)
- Diced red onion (1)
- Beetroots (8)
- Balsamic vinegar (4 sp.)
- Chutney (80ml)
- Mayo (80ml0

How's it done

1. Add the beetroot and water to a pan and let it boil, cooking the beetroot for 20 minutes. Wash with cold water and remove the skin before slicing.
2. Mix the beetroot and onion together.
3. Now work on the dressing. Add the balsamic vinegar, mayo, and chutney together.
4. Take out a platter and add the vegetables and pour the dressing on top. Garnish with the onion and pecans and serve over feta cheese.

Nutrition
Calories: 413
Fat: 31.9g
Carbs: 28.2g
Protein: 7.2g

Salmon and Potato Salad

Prep time: 10 minutes
Cooking time: 25 minutes
Servings: 6

What's in it

- Chopped parsley (1 Tbsp.)
- Salmon (6 oz.)
- Chopped onion (1)
- Olive oil (1 Tbsp.)
- Baking potatoes (3)

How's it done

1. Boil the potatoes and eggs together until done. While those are boiling, heat up some oil in a pan and fry the onions.
2. Place the salmon slices into a dish and put the onions on top.
3. Top with the eggs and he potatoes and sprinkle the parsley on top before serving.

Nutrition
Calories: 400
Fat: 30g
Carbs: 10g
Protein: 15g

Smoked Salmon

Prep time: 10 minutes
Cooking time: 0 minutes
Servings: 4

What's in it

- Salmon caviar (2 Tbsp.)
- Olive oil (1 Tbsp.)
- Pepper
- Creamed horseradish (1 Tbsp.)
- Lemon zest (1)
- Greek yogurt (100g)
- Cream cheese (200g.)
- Smoked salmon (100g)

How's it done

1. Take out your food blender and add the Greek yogurt, cream cheese, salmon, and lemon zest.
2. Add in the pepper and horseradish as well. Blend these together until nice and smooth.
3. Put this into a bowl and drizzle on the olive oil and salmon caviar and serve.

Nutrition
Calories: 318
Fat: 26g
Carbs: 2g
Protein: 14g

Burgers for Lunch

Prep time: 5 minutes
Cooking time: 15 minutes
Servings: 3

What's in it

- Sliced onion (4 slices)
- Olive oil (2 Tbsp.)
- Pepper (1 pinch)
- Salt (1 pinch)
- Steak seasoning (1 Tbsp.)
- Worcestershire sauce (1 Tbsp.)
- Beef (1 lb.)

How's it done

1. Mix the steak seasoning, Worcestershire sauce, and beef together. Form into patties.
2. Sprinkle each with some pepper and salt. Bring out a skillet and fry the onions with the oil until they turn an amber color.
3. Add the patties to the skillet and cook until they reach the desired doneness. Top with the caramelized onions and serve.

Nutrition
Calories: 479
Fat: 40g
Carbs: 2g
Protein: 26g

Blue Bison Burgers

Prep time: 20 minutes
Cooking time: 10 minutes
Servings: 4

What's in it

- Garlic cloves (2)
- Salt
- Pepper (1 tsp.)
- Worcestershire sauce (2 Tbsp.)
- Blue cheese (.25 lb.)
- Bacon (.5 lb.)
- Ground chuck (.5 lb.)
- Ground bison (2 lbs.)

How's it done

1. Grind the bacon in a blender to make them crumbly. Then add these to a bowl with the remainder of the ingredients.
2. Form this into patties and then place on the preheated grill. Cook until they reach desired doneness.
3. Top with lettuce leaves and enjoy.

Nutrition
Calories: 708
Fat: 59g
Carbs: 10g
Protein: 34g

Blue Cheese Salad

Prep time: 10 minutes
Cooking time: 10 minutes
Servings: 1

What's in it

- Blue cheese (.25 c.)
- Bacon (4 pieces)
- Steak seasoning (3 Tbsp.)
- Beef (1 lb.)
- Pepper
- Salt
- Olive oil (4 Tbsp.)
- Lemon juice (2 Tbsp.)
- Lettuce head (1)
- Red pepper (1)

How's it done

1. Take out a skillet and brown the beef. Add in the steak seasoning.
2. In a second skillet, cook up the bacon until done.
3. Create the dressing by mixing the pepper, salt, olive oil, and lemon juice. Mix with the red pepper.
4. Place the dressing on a plate and top with the cooked beef. Add more on top and then top with the bacon and blue cheese.

Nutrition
Calories: 747
Fat: 4.7g
Carbs: 11.6g
Protein: 41.7g

Red Salad

Prep time: 5 minutes
Cooking time: 0 minutes
Servings: 6

What's in it

- Garlic clove (1)
- Lemon juice (1 Tbsp.)
- Butter milk (4 Tbsp.)
- Sour cream (4 Tbsp.)
- Peppadew peppers (60g)
- Sliced onion (1)
- Sliced radishes (8)
- Red kidney beans (400g)
- Chopped coriander (2 Tbsp)
- Sugar (.5 tsp.)
- Micro herbs (35g)

How's it done

1. Spread the onion, peppers, radishes, and kidneys on a platter.
2. Make the dressing by combining the rest of the ingredients together.
3. Pour this on top of the vegetable sin the platter and then serve.

Nutrition
Calories: 55
Fat: .8g
Carbs: 10.2g
Protein: 2.1g

Black Beans and Rice

Prep time: 5 minutes
Cooking time: 20 minutes
Servings: 10

What's in it

- Black beans (3.5 c.)
- Pepper
- Cumin (1 tsp.)
- Vegetable broth (1.5 c.)
- White rice (.75 c.)
- Garlic cloves (2)
- Onion (1)
- Olive oil (1 tsp.)

How's it done

1. Heat up some oil in a pan. Add the garlic and onions to fry. When those are warm, add in the rice and cook a few more minutes.
2. After this time, add in the vegetable broth and let the rice cook with the lid on.
3. Add in the rest of the ingredients and then serve warm.

Nutrition
Calories: 140
Fat: .9g
Carbs: 27.1g
Protein: 6.3g

Barley and Mushroom Soup

Prep time: 25 minutes
Cooking time: 30 minutes
Servings: 6

What's in it

- Vegetable broth (5 c.)
- Mushrooms (20 oz.)
- Celery stalks (2)
- Carrot (1)
- Pepper and salt
- Onions (2)
- Olive oil (1.5 Tbsp.)
- Barley (1 c.)
- Bay leaves (2)
- Thyme (2 Tbsp.)

How's it done

1. Boil the barley with four cups of water. While that is heating up, heat some oil in a pan and add the onion, salt, and peppers.
2. Now add in the celery and carrots and cook or a few minutes before adding in the rest of the ingredients and cook for another 10 minutes.
3. Add in the barley and cook a few more minutes. Serve warm.

Nutrition
Calories: 194
Fat: 4.9g
Carbs: 20g
Protein: 9.6g

Chapter 6
Dinner Ideas for the Whole Family

Pumpkin Soup

Prep time: 20 minutes
Cooking time: 50 minutes
Servings: 6

What's in it

- Pumpkin (3 lbs.)
- Pumpkin seeds (.25 c.)
- Water (1 c.)
- Crushed garlic clove (1)
- Salt (1 tsp.)
- Coconut cream (2 c.)
- Butter (2 Tbsp.)
- Chopped onion (1)
- Olive oil (.25 c.)

How's it done

1. Allow the oven to heat up to 400 degrees. Take the pulp and seeds out of the pumpkin and chop up into cubes.
2. Place the pumpkin on a tray and drizzle on the olive oil. Place in the oven and cook for 40 minutes.
3. While the pumpkin is baking, cook the butter and chopped onion together until it is soft.
4. Add the cream to a bowl and blend so it becomes whipped. Add the salt, garlic, and onion ad blend.
5. Take the pumpkin out of the oven and let it cool. Then remove the skin and add the flesh

to your other ingredients. Blend until smooth.
6. Warm up in a pan, adding some water to make it as thin as you would like. Add the seeds on top and serve.

Nutrition
Calories: 500
Fats: 30g
Carbs: 18g
Protein: 6g

Super Green Soup

Prep time: 5 minutes
Cooking time: 20 minutes
Servings: 6

What's in it

- Pepper
- Salt
- Coconut oil (.25 c.)
- Coconut milk (1 c.)
- Vegetable stock (1 liter)
- Spinach (2 c.)
- Watercress (1 c.)
- Bay leaf (1)
- Minced garlic cloves (2)
- Chopped onion (1)
- Chopped cauliflower head (1)

How's it done

1. Grease up a pan with some oil and cook the garlic and onion. When those are browned, add the bay leaf and cauliflower and cook for another 5 minutes.
2. Add the spinach and watercress and cook for a bit to wilt. Pour in the vegetable stock and let this boil. Cook for another 8 minutes.
3. Add in the coconut milk and then remove from the heat. Blend so this becomes smooth and creamy.
4. This can be frozen or left in the fridge for five days.

Nutrition
Calories: 392   Fats: 38g

Carbs: 7g   Protein: 5g
Beof Stew

Prep time: 5 minutes
Cooking time: 8 hours
Servings: 7

What's in it

- Salt
- Worcestershire sauce (1 Tbsp.)
- Hot chili sauce (2 tsp.)
- Beef broth (1 c.)
- Chili mix (1 Tbsp.)
- Chopped tomatoes (2 cans)
- Stew beef, cubed (1.5 lbs.)

How's it done

1. Take out the slow cooker and turn it on a low setting.
2. Add all of the ingredients inside and mix around. Cook this mixture for eight hours before serving.

Nutrition
Calories: 222
Fats: 7g
Carbs: 9g
Protein: 27g

Vegetable Dinner

Prep time: 5 minutes
Cooking time: 20 minutes
Servings: 1

What's in it

- Sliced orange pepper (.25)
- Sliced green pepper (.25)
- Sliced red pepper (.25)
- Sliced onion (.5)
- Chopped cauliflower (1 head)
- Olive oil (1 Tbsp.)
- Eggs (2)
- Dill

How's it done

1. Heat up some oil in a skillet or a pan. Place half an inch of water in a bowl and add the cauliflower. Cook in the microwave for four minutes.
2. When the oil is hot, fry the onions and pepper for a few minutes. Add in a few tablespoons of water as needed.
3. Add in the seasonings and the cauliflower and cook this for another ten minutes.
4. Add in the eggs and cook at this time as well. Add to some lettuce leaves and serve.

Nutrition
Calories: 145
Fats: 12g
Carbs: 3g
Protein: 12g

Bacon Burgers

Prep time: 10 minutes
Cooking time: 60 minutes
Servings: 12

What's in it

- Pepper
- Salt
- Onion powder (1 pinch)
- Cumin powder (1 pinch)
- Raw sausage patties (121
- 1-inch cubes of cheddar cheese
- Bacon (12 slices)

How's it done

1. Allow the oven to heat up to 350 degrees. Line a baking tray with some parchment paper. Add the sausage patties to this tray.
2. Add the seasonings to the sausage and then place a piece of the cheese in the middle of the patties. Wrap the sausage around the cheese into a ball.
3. Add the baking pan into the oven. After an hour, take them out and let cool down.

Nutrition
Calories: 250
Fats: 20g
Carbs: 1g
Protein: 14g

Italian Meatballs

Prep time: 5 minutes
Cooking time: 40 minutes
Servings: 4

What's in it

- Dried thyme (1 tsp.)
- Dried oregano (1 tsp.)
- Sliced mozzarella (.5 c.)
- Peeled tomatoes (1 can)
- Minced beef (1 lb.)
- Basil (1 handful)
- Tomato paste (1 Tbsp.)
- Crushed garlic cloves (2)
- Red onion, diced (.5 c.)

How's it done

1. Allow the oven to heat up to 350 degrees. Take out a bowl and mix together the ground beef and herbs. Form into 16 meatballs.
2. Fry these in a skillet for five minutes to make them brown. Take a bit of the cooking juices and set to the side.
3. Add the garlic, tomato paste, onion, and tinned tomatoes into the ban. Simmer this for another ten minutes.
4. Place the meatballs into a dish and top with this sauce. Break up the cheese and spread it on the tomato sauce.
5. Cover the dish with some foil and place in the oven. Bake for 20 minutes. Take the foil off and bake a bit longer.
6. Serve with a salad.

Nutrition

Calories: 380   Fats: 23g

Carbs: 8g   Protein: 25g
Beef Welly

Prep time: 20 minutes
Cooking time: 20 minutes
Servings: 2

What's in it

- Almond flour (.5 c.)
- Mozzarella cheese (1 c.)
- Liver pate (4 Tbsp.)
- Butter (1 Tbsp.)
- Tenderloin steaks (2)

How's it done

1. Season the steaks. Melt some butter in a pan and let it heat up before adding the steaks to the pan. Sear it on all sides and then let them cool down.
2. Heat up some mozzarella in the microwave for a minute. Add in the almond flour to form a dough.
3. Place this dough between two pieces of parchment paper and the roll it flat. Place some pate on the dough and spread it out.
4. Cut the dough so that it can make a ball around the meat. Add some meat into the dough and cut it, wrapping it around the meat. Do this with the other piece of meat as well.
5. Allow the oven to heat up to 400 degrees. Place into the oven and let it bake. After 20 minutes, it is done.

Nutrition
Calories: 307   Fats: 22g

Carbs: 2.5g   Protein: 26g

Salmon Fishcakes

Prep time: 12 minutes
Cooking time: 12 minutes
Servings: 2

What's in it

- Hollandaise sauce (1 jar)
- Pepper
- Salt
- Chives (2 Tbsp.)
- Butter (.5 Tbsp.)
- Sliced salmon (4 oz.)
- Eggs (2)

How's it done

1. Take the time to hard-boil your eggs. Dice up the salmon while the eggs cook.
2. Take out a skillet and heat up some butter at a high heat. Place half the salmon inside and crisp it up before setting aside.
3. Run the prepared eggs under some cold water and peel. Mash them into a fine piece.
4. Take the raw salmon and half the chives and mix with the egg, along with a few tablespoons of the Hollandaise sauce.
5. Split this into four lumps and turn into balls.
6. Mix the crispy salmon and chives together and dip the egg balls into them until coated.

Nutrition
Calories: 295
Fats: 23g
Carbs: 1g
Protein: 18g

Garlic Pork Chops

Prep time: 5 minutes
Cooking time: 15 minutes
Servings: 4

What's in it

- Chopped onion (.75)
- Crushed garlic (1 tsp.)
- Paprika (1 Tbsp.)
- Pork chops (4)
- Chopped parsley (1 Tbsp.)
- Heavy cream (.5 c.)
- Butter (1 Tbsp.)
- Sliced mushrooms (1 c.)
- Coconut oil (2 Tbsp.)
- Cayenne pepper (.25 tsp.)
- Salt (1 tsp.)
- Pepper (1 tsp.)

How's it done

1. Mix together the seasonings with a third of the onion. Sprinkle on both chops and rub it in.
2. Heat up some coconut oil and brown the chops for a few minutes on both sides. Set them to the side.
3. Add in the rest of the mushrooms and onions and cook another four minutes to make the onions clear.
4. In a new pan, whisk the butter and cream on a low heat. Place the chops into the cream sauce and cook for another five minutes.

Nutrition
Calories: 481   Fats: 32g

Carbs: 4g   Protein: 15g
Spaghetti Carbonara

Prep time: 4 minutes
Cooking time: 20 minutes
Servings: 4

What's in it

- Shirataki noodles (3 packets)
- Chopped bacon (5 oz.)
- Butter (1.5 Tbsp.)
- Garlic cloves (2)
- Grated cheese (1 c.)
- Eggs (3)

How's it done

1. Melt the butter in a pan and then add the bacon and cook until crispy. Then add in the noodles and the garlic.
2. Stir the noodles as they are heating up. While those are cooking, bring out a new bowl and beat the eggs with some of the cheese.
3. Add the cooked noodles to a new bowl. Stir the egg and cheese mixture into this, watching for the sauce to thicken.
4. Top with the parsley and the rest of the cheese and enjoy.

Nutrition
Calories: 361
Fats: 29g
Carbs: 4.5g
Protein: 16g

Shrimp Tuscany

Prep time: 0 minutes
Cooking time: 15 minutes
Servings: 4

What's in it

- Baby kale (.25 c.)
- Sun dried tomatoes (5)
- Parmesan (.5 c.)
- Salt (1 tsp.)
- Dried basil (1 tsp.)
- Crushed garlic cloves (2)
- Whole milk (.5 c.)
- Cream cheese, cubed (1 c.)
- Butter (1 Tbsp.)
- Raw shrimp (1 lb.)

How's it done

1. Melt up the butter in a pan and add in the shrimp. Cook for 30 seconds and then turn them around. Cook until they turn pink.
2. Add in the cream cheese and milk into the pan and increase the heat. Stir so the cheese melts completely.
3. Add in the basil, salt, and garlic and keep cooking. Allow the dish to simmer so that the sauce can thicken.
4. Add in the tomatoes and kale and then serve.

Nutrition
Calories: 298
Fats: 18g
Carbs: 6.5g
Protein: 23g

Sea Bass

Prep time: 15 minutes
Cooking time: 15 minutes
Servings: 2

What's in it

- Lemons (2)
- Green olives (.3 c.)
- Grated cauliflower (1 c.)
- Sea bass (1)
- Pepper
- Salt
- Chopped parsley (.33 c.)
- Chopped mint (.33 c.)

How's it done

1. Allow the oven to heat up to 400 degrees. Place some parchment paper on a baking pan and place the fish on top. Add some oil to the fish.
2. Slice the lemons and stuff into the bass along with the herbs. Place into the oven to bake for 15 minutes.
3. Chop up the olives and juice the other lemons. Take out a bowl and mix together the rest of the ingredients.
4. Serve the prepare fish with the cauliflower salad.

Nutrition
Calories: 380
Fats: 26g
Carbs: 3.4g
Protein: 27g

Eggs and Bacon

Prep time: 5 minutes
Cooking time: 15 minutes
Servings: 6

What's in it

- Pepper
- Salt
- Paprika (.75 tsp.)
- Mustard (1.5 Tbsp.)
- Mayo (2.25 Tbsp.)
- Chopped bacon slices (6)
- Eggs, hard boiled (9)

How's it done

1. Take out a skillet and heat it up to cook the bacon until crisp. Move to a plate with some paper towels to drain.
2. Halve the eggs and scoop out the yolks. Arrange the halves on a plater. Mash the yolks with the paprika, mayo, salt, pepper, and mustard.
3. Dice the bacon and then add some into the yolk mixture to stir well.
4. Spoon the yolk back into the egg whites and divide the rest of the bacon among them. Serve or store.

Nutrition
Calories: 283
Fats: 21g
Carbs: 3g
Protein: 20g

Caesar Salad

Prep time: 15 minutes
Cooking time: 0 minutes
Servings: 6

What's in it

- Garlic powder (.33 tsp.)
- Anchovy paste (.33 tsp.)
- Mayo (1.5 Tbsp.)
- Lemon juice (3 Tbsp.)
- Parmesan cheese (.33 c.)
- Olive oil (.33 c.)
- Chopped romaine lettuce (12 c.)

How's it done

1. Combine the mayo, garlic powder, anchovy paste, olive oil, and lemon juice. Whisk well and divide into 6 servings.
2. In a bowl, toss the cheese and the lettuce. Divide between six containers and enjoy.

Nutrition
Calories: 93
Fats: 7g
Carbs: 6g
Protein: 3g

Cheesy Avocado Wedges

Prep time: 5 minutes
Cooking time: 10 minutes
Servings: 4

What's in it

- Pepper
- Salt
- Onion powder (.33 tsp.)
- Garlic powder (.33 tsp.)
- Heavy cream (1.5 Tbsp.)
- Parmesan cheese (.33 c.)
- Ground pork rinds (.33 c.)
- Avocado (1)
- Eggs (2)

How's it done

1. Place a skillet on the stove and add a bit of oil. Heat up the oil nice and hot.
2. Take out a bowl and whisk the eggs and mix to make smooth. Halve the avocado and then scoop out the flesh before slicing. Season with pepper and salt.
3. Take out a plate and combine the garlic powder, onion powder, pork rinds, and Parmesan.
4. Add the avocado to the egg mixture and then dredge into the cheese mixture. Add these to the hot oil and cook for a minute on each side.
5. Move to a platter and drain before storing or serving.

Nutrition
Calories: 179   Fats: 14g

Carbs: 6g   Protein: 8g

Beef Chili

Prep time: 15 minutes
Cooking time: 1 hour
Servings: 3

What's in it

- Garlic powder (.25 tsp.)
- Cumin seeds (.5 tsp.)
- Dried oregano (1 tsp.)
- Chili powder (1 Tbsp.)
- Flaxseed meal (2 Tbsp.)
- Olive oil (.25 c.)
- Beef broth (2 c.)
- Ground beef (1 lb.)
- Diced yellow onion (1)

How's it done

1. Take out a pot and heat it up on the stove. Add in the onion and beef and cook the beef through.
2. Stir in the rest of the ingredients and bring it all to a boil. Let this cook for an hour, stirring the whole time.
3. After this time. take the chili from the heat and allow it to cool before storing.

Nutrition
Calories: 567
Fats: 36g
Carbs: 18g
Protein: 41g

Garlic Cod

Prep time: 5 minutes
Cooking time: 20 minutes
Servings: 3

What's in it

- Pepper
- Salt
- Minced garlic (1.5 Tbsp.)
- Sliced butter (.33 c.)
- Baby bok choy (.75 lb.)
- Cod fillets (3)

How's it done

1. Allow the oven to heat up to 400 degrees. Cut out 3 sheets of foil and use each one to cover the fillets. Place the fillets on these and add the garlic and butter.
2. Add the bok choy and then season. Fold over the pouches and place onto a baking sheet. Place into the oven.
3. After 20 minutes, take them out of the oven and let them cool down before storing.

Nutrition
Calories: 355
Fats: 21g
Carbs: 3g
Protein: 37g

Chicken Soup

Prep time: 15 minutes
Cooking time: 20 minutes
Serving: 4

What's in it

- Olive oil (.25 c.)
- Diced carrot (.25 c,)
- Diced celery (.5 c.)
- Water (.5 c.)
- Macadamia nuts (.5 c.)
- Chicken breast, cooked and diced
- Chicken broth (2 c.)
- Diced yellow onion (1)

How's it done

1. Take out a pan and heat it up. Add in the oil and swirl to coat around. Cook the celery, onion, and carrot together.
2. Stir in the chicken broth and the macadamia nuts. Bring this to a simmer until the carrots are tender.
3. Turn the heat off and let this cool down. Take out the immersion blender and blend to make smooth. Pour into the pan.
4. Add half a cup to the soup and stir. Heat it back up and add the chicken back in. ladle it up or store.

Nutrition
Calories: 325
Fats: 28g
Carbs: 7g
Protein: 14g

Ginger Sesame Halibut

Prep time: 20 minutes
Cooking time: 20 minutes
Servings: 3

What's in it

- Rice wine vinegar (.75 tsp.)
- Sesame oil (.75 tsp.)
- Olive oil (1.5 tsp.)
- Soy sauce (1.5 tsp.)
- Minced ginger (1.5 Tbsp.)
- Alaskan Halibut fillets (3)

How's it done

1. Allow the oven to heat up to 400 degrees. Add some foil to a baking sheet and set aside.
2. Take out a bowl and combine the olive and sesame oil. Then add in the ginger, soy sauce, and rice vinegar.
3. Add the fish into the bowl and turn to coat. Arrange on the baking sheet and place in oven.
4. Bake for 17 minutes to cook the fish. Allow them to cool down and then place in the fridge.

Nutrition
Calories: 237
Fats: 35g
Carbs: 1g
Protein: 33g

Coconut Chicken

Prep time: 5 minutes
Cooking time: 7 minutes
Servings: 4

What's in it

- Coconut oil (1 Tbsp.)
- Coconut milk (8 oz.)
- Water (.25 c.)
- Salt
- Pepper
- Chicken thighs (1 lb.)
- Apple cider vinegar (4 Tbsp.)
- Garlic cloves (5)

How's it done

1. Take out a pan and heat up the coconut oil inside. Add in the chicken thighs and cook for a few minutes.
2. Add in the garlic cloves and the apple vinegar. Season with the pepper and salt.
3. Add in the coconut milk and cook a bit longer before serving.

Nutrition
Calories: 286
Fat: 20g
Carbs: 3g
Protein: 23g

Grilled Chicken Skewers

Prep time: 15 minutes
Cooking time: 10 minutes
Servings: 2

What's in it

- Olive oil (1 c.)
- Salt
- Lemon juice (.25 c.)
- Garlic clove (1)
- Zucchini (1)
- Bell peppers, chopped (2)
- Chopped onion (1)
- Chicken breast, cubed (1 lb.)

How's it done

1. Work on the sauce first. To do this, mix together the olive oil, lemon juice, salt, and garlic clove. Add the chicken to half the sauce and reserve the rest.
2. Add the zucchini, peppers, and onion in to marinate as well.
3. After marinating, place on skewers and then grill the ingredients until done. Serve warm.

Nutrition
Calories: 580
Fat: 21g
Carbs: 11g
Protein: 55g

Garlic Cod

Prep time: 5 minutes
Cooking time:
Servings: 4

What's in it

- Salt (1 pinch)
- Garlic powder (1 Tbsp.)
- Garlic cloves (6)
- Ghee (3 Tbsp.)
- Cod fillets (4)

How's it done

1. Take out a frying pan and melt the ghee on it. Then add the garlic and fry it up.
2. When the garlic is warm, add in the cod fillets and sprinkle on the garlic powder and the salt.
3. Flip the cod around and cook for a few minutes before serving.

Nutrition

Calories: 160
Fat: 7g
Carbs: 4g
Protein: 21g

Lamb Chops

Prep time: 10 minutes
Cooking time: 6 minutes
Servings: 6

What's in it

- Lamb chops (2 lbs.)
- Olive oil (2 Tbsp.)
- Sliced onion (1)
- Minced garlic (1 Tbsp.)
- Pepper
- Salt (2 tsp.)
- Vinegar (.25 c.)

How's it done

1. Take out a bowl and mix together the olive oil, onion, garlic, pepper, salt, and vinegar.
2. Add the lamb chops into this and let it marinate for ten minutes.
3. After this time, heat up the grill and place the lamp chops on there. Cook for three minutes on both sides and then serve.

Nutrition
Calories: 519
Fat: 44.8g
Carbs: 2.3g
Protein: 25g

Flourless Pizza

Prep time: 10 minutes
Cooking time: 15 minutes
Servings: 2

What's in it

- Pepper
- Salt
- Shredded cheese (.33 c.)
- Tomato sauce (.33 c.)
- Olive oil (1 Tbsp.)
- Parmesan cheese (.5 c.)
- Sliced eggplant (.5)

How's it done

1. Allow the oven to heat up to 375 degrees. Add the eggplant to a baking tray and drizzle the oil and cheese on top. Place into the oven.
2. After the cheese has melted, take out of the oven and scoop the sauce on top. Place back into the oven to bake a little longer.
3. Serve with some pepper and salt on top.

Nutrition
Calories: 274
Fat: 19.1g
Carbs: 13g
Protein: 14.6g

Chapter 7
Snacks to Fill Your Hunger

Cream Cheese Cucumber Bites

Prep time: 15 minutes
Cooking time: 0 minutes
Servings: 5

What's in it

- Tabasco sauce
- Chopped green onion (.5 Tbsp.)
- Lemon juice (1 Tbsp.)
- Flaked red salmon (4 oz.)
- Cream cheese (8 oz.)
- Avocado (1)
- Sliced cucumber (1)

How's it done

1. Halve the avocado and get rid of the stone. Scoop out the flesh and place into a bowl. Mash the avocado and cream cheese to make smooth.
2. Add in the lemon juice and season with the tabasco sauce. Arrange the cucumber on a platter.
3. Divide up the avocado mixture on top of them. divide up the salmon on top as well and then serve.

Nutrition
Calories: 277
Fats: 22g
Carbs: 5g

Protein: 19g

Ham and Cheese Puffs

Prep time: 15 minutes
Cooking time: 30 minutes
Servings: 9

What's in it

- Baking soda (.33 tsp.)
- Baking powder (.33 tsp.)
- Coconut oil (.33 c.)
- Coconut flour (.33 c.)
- Mayo (.75 c.)
- Cheddar cheese (1.5 c.)
- Diced deli ham (10 oz.)
- Eggs (6)

How's it done

1. Allow the oven to heat up to 350 degrees. Prepare a baking sheet.
2. Take out a bowl and mix together the mayo, coconut oil, and eggs. Set this to the side.
3. In another bowl, combine the coconut flour, baking powder, and baking soda. Combine the two mixtures together. Fold in the cheddar and ham and set aside.
4. Divide the dough into 18 pieces and arrange on the baking sheet. Place into the oven.
5. Bake these for 30 minutes. Take them out of the oven and allow them to cool down before storing.

Nutrition

Calories: 249   Fats: 20g
Carbs: 3g   Protein:15g

Walnut Bites

Prep time: 10 minutes
Cooking time: 8 minutes
Servings: 10

What's in it

- Chopped thyme (.5 Tbsp.)
- Butter (1 Tbsp.)
- Chopped walnuts (2 Tbsp.)
- Parmesan cheese (6 oz.)

How's it done

1. Allow the oven to heat up to 350 degrees. Line two baking sheets.
2. Take out a food processor and combine the butter and Parmesan cheese. Pour in the walnuts and process until combined.
3. Use a tablespoon to scoop this mixture onto the baking sheet. Top with the thyme. Place into the oven.
4. Bake these for eight minutes and then cool down before storing or eating.

Nutrition
Calories: 80
Fats: 3g
Carbs: 7g
Protein: 7g

Smoked Salmon and Dill Spread

Prep time: 20 minutes
Cooking time: 0 minutes
Servings: 8

What's in it

- Salt
- Pepper
- Chopped dill (2 Tbsp.)
- Mayo (2.5 Tbsp.)
- Cream cheese (4 oz)
- Smoked salmon (4 oz.)

How's it done

1. Pour the cream cheese, mayo, and salmon into a food processor to combine.
2. Pour this into a container to store it and mix in the salt, pepper, and dill.
3. Store it properly.

Nutrition
Calories: 70
Fats: 5g
Carbs: 2g
Protein: 5g

Lime and Coconut Fat Bombs

Prep time: 1 hr. 15 minutes
Cooking time: 0 minutes
Servings: 8

What's in it

- Liquid stevia (.5 tsp.)
- Lime extract (.5 tsp.)
- Lime juice (1 Tbsp.)
- Heavy cream (2 Tbsp.)
- Coconut oil (2 Tbsp.)
- Butter (2 Tbsp.)
- Cream cheese (1 oz.)

How's it done

1. Combine the butter, coconut oil, and cream cheese into a bowl. Microwave until melted.
2. Stir this mixture and add in the cream. Mix before adding in the rest of the ingredients.
3. Take out an ice cube tray and pour the mixture inside. Freeze for an hour and then store.

Nutrition
Calories: 81
Fats: 9g
Carbs: .4g
Protein: .4g

Chocolate and Peanut Fat Bombs

Prep time: 1 hr. 15 minutes
Cooking time: 0 minutes
Servings: 8

What's in it

- Liquid stevia (.5 tsp.)
- Vanilla (.5 tsp.)
- Cocoa powder (1 Tbsp.)
- Peanut butter (1 Tbsp.)
- Heavy cream (2 Tbsp.)
- Coconut oil (2 Tbsp.)
- Butter (2 Tbsp.)

How's it done

1. Combine the butter, coconut oil, and peanut butter in a bowl. Microwave until melted.
2. Stir the mixture before adding in the rest of your ingredients.
3. Pour this mixture into an ice cube tray with eight compartments. Place into the freezer for an hour. Store or serve.

Nutrition
Calories: 73
Fats: 8g
Carbs: 1g
Protein: .6g

Almond and Herb Tapenade

Prep time: 15 minutes
Cooking time: 0 minutes
Servings: 8

What's in it

- Salt
- Drained capers (.5 tsp.)
- Lemon juice (.5 Tbsp.)
- Olive oil (.25 c.)
- Basil leaves (.25 c.)
- Slivered almonds (.25 c.)
- Pitted green olives (1 c.)
- Minced garlic cloves

How's it done

1. Take out the food processor and combine the lemon juice, capers, olives, garlic, and almonds. Add in the basil leaves and pulse some more.
2. Pour in the salt and olive oil. Pulse to make this into a paste.
3. Add this to a container and store well.

Nutrition
Calories: 28
Fats: 3g
Carbs: .36g
Protein: .1g

Chocolate Bacon

Prep time: 15 minutes
Cooking time: 20 minutes
Servings: 6

What's in it

- Liquid stevia (1.5 tsp.)
- Coconut oil (2.25 Tbsp.)
- Dark chocolate (4.5 Tbsp.)
- Bacon slices (12)

How's it done

1. Allow the oven to heat up to 425 degrees. Skewer the bacon on some iron skewers and place on a baking sheet. Add into the oven.
2. After 15 minutes, take the bacon out and allow it to cool.
3. Melt the coconut oil in a pan before stirring in the chocolate. Let the chocolate melt and add the stevia as well.
4. Place the bacon onto some parchment paper and coat with the chocolate on both sides. Allow the chocolate to dry and then serve.

Nutrition
Calories: 258
Fats: 26g
Carbs: .5g
Protein: 7g

Cinnamon Butter

Prep time: 10 minutes
Cooking time: 0 minutes
Servings: 8

What's in it

- Salt
- Cinnamon (.5 tsp.)
- Vanilla (.5 tsp.)
- Liquid stevia (5 drops)
- Butter (.5 c.)

How's it done

1. Combine the stevia, salt, cinnamon, vanilla, and butter. Mix to make smooth.
2. Add some wax paper on a baking sheet and spread this mixture on top. Roll up the paper and seal the ends.
3. Place in the fridge for an hour before using.

Nutrition
Calories: 103
Fats: 12g
Carbs: .1g
Protein: .1g

Cheddar Bites

Prep time: 15 minutes
Cooking time: 1 hour and 30 minutes
Servings: 6

What's in it

- Paprika
- Pepper
- Salt
- Butter (2 Tbsp.)
- Heavy cream (2 Tbsp.)
- Cheddar cheese (.5 c.)
- Egg whites (4)
- Cauliflower (1)

How's it done

1. Add the cauliflower into a pot with a bit of water. Season with some salt. Bring this to a high simmer and cook to make the cauliflower tender.
2. Drain out and add the cauliflower with the cream and butter to the food processor and make it combine.
3. Beat the egg whites to get soft peaks to form. Fold in the cauliflower mixture to combine and then add in the cheddar cheese.
4. Cover the bowl and leave this in the fridge for 30 minutes.
5. Allow the oven to heat up to 375 degrees. Scoop the mixture onto a baking sheet and place into the oven.
6. After 30 minutes take these out and let them cool before storing.

Nutrition

Calories: 142   Fats: 10g
Carbs: 7g   Protein: 8g

Bacon and Mozzarella Sticks

Prep time: 10 minutes
Cooking time: 5 minutes
Servings: 4

What's in it

- Sunflower oil
- Mozzarella string cheese (4 pieces)
- Bacon strips (8)

How's it done

1. Heat up some oil in a skillet. While that heats up, halve the string cheese and wrap with the bacon.
2. Cook these in the oil for a few minutes to brown the bacon.
3. Add these on a plate with the paper towels and let it drain. Store well.

Nutrition
Calories: 278
Fats: 15g
Carbs: 3g
Protein: 32g

Garlicky Corn

Prep time: 5 minutes
Cooking time: 10 minutes
Servings: 2

What's in it

- Pepper
- Salt
- Butter (2 Tbsp.)
- Parsley (1 Tbsp.)
- Zucchini (2 c.)
- Yellow squash (2 c.)
- Corn (1 cob)
- Vegetable broth (.5 c.)
- Onion (.5)
- Olive oil (2 Tbsp.)

How's it done

1. Heat up some oil in a pan and cook the garlic and onion for a few minutes.
2. Next, add in the zucchini, squash, corn, and vegetable broth and cook to make these warm.
3. Mix in the butter and the parsley and season with salt and pepper before serving.

Nutrition
Calories: 178
Fat: 12.6g
Carbs: 17.1g
Protein: 3g

Avocado Toast

Prep time:10 minutes
Cooking time: 5 minutes
Servings: 2

What's in it

- Peeled avocado (1)
- Cheddar cheese (2 oz.)
- Bread slices (2)

How's it done

1. Allow the oven to heat up to 300 degrees. Top your bread slices with the cheese and add to the oven.
2. Let this cook until the cheese melts. Top with the avocado slices and then serve.

Nutrition
Calories: 72
Fat: 1.2g
Carbs: 5.2g
Protein: 3.6g

Coleslaw

Prep time: 20 minutes
Cooking time: 0 minutes
Servings: 14

What's in it

- Lemon juice (1 Tbsp.)
- Balsamic vinegar (.3 c.)
- Olive oil (.66 c.)
- Onion (1)
- Carrots (2)
- Shredded red cabbage (.5)
- Shredded cabbage head (1)
- Shredded kale (1 bunch)
- Maple syrup (1 tsp.)

How's it done

1. Take out a bowl and mix together the vegetables. In a second bowl, whisk together the remainder of the ingredients.
2. Drizzle this dressing on the vegetables and mix to coat. Place into the fridge until ready to eat.

Nutrition
Calories: 91
Fat: 4.1g
Carbs: 13g
Protein: 2.3g

Mexican Coleslaw

Prep time: 15 minutes
Cooking time: 0 minutes
Servings: 8

What's in it

- Pepper
- Salt
- Chopped cilantro (.3 c.)
- Olive oil (.2 Tbsp.)
- Rice vinegar (.25 c.)
- Carrots (1.5 c.)
- Sliced green cabbage (6)

How's it done

1. Rinse the carrots and cabbage in cold water and then add to a bowl. In a second bowl, make your dressing by mixing the remainder of the ingredients.
2. Drizzle the dressing over the vegetables and toss to coat. Leave in the fridge for up to a day before eating.

Nutrition
Calories: 52
Fat: 3.5g
Carbs: 5.1g
Protein: 1g

Chapter 8
Desserts to End the Day

Coconut Macaroons

Prep time: 2 hours and 20 minutes
Cooking time: 0 minutes
Servings: 18

What's in it

- Stevia (2.25 tsp.)
- Coconut milk (.75 c.)
- Shredded coconut (1.5 c.)

How's it done

1. Combine together the ingredients in a bowl, mixing well.
2. Pack this down with some plastic wrap and then place in the fridge for a few hours.
3. Once it is chilled, scoop the mixture into balls and then place in a container to store.

Nutrition
Calories: 47
Fats: 5g
Carbs: 2g
Protein: .4g

Raspberry Pops

Prep time: 20 minutes
Cooking time: 0 minutes
Servings: 8

What's in it

- Vanilla (1 tsp.)
- Butter (4 Tbsp.)
- Heavy cream (4 Tbsp.)
- Coconut oil (4 Tbsp.)
- Chopped raspberries (.25 c.)
- Cream cheese (.25 c.)

How's it done

1. Mix the butter, coconut oil, and cream cheese together. Microwave these to melt.
2. Take the bowl out of the microwave and stir around. Add in the heavy cream and fold the raspberries.
3. Stir the vanilla and make sure to combine well. Take out an ice cube tray with 16 sections and put into the freezer.
4. Let these chill until frozen.

Nutrition
Calories: 166
Fats: 17g
Carbs: 2g
Protein: .8g

Coco Peanut Butter Bites

Prep time: 15 minutes
Cooking time: 12 minutes
Servings: 12

What's in it

- Coconut flour (3 tsp.)
- Stevia (4.5 tsp.)
- Butter (.75 c.)
- Peanut butter (.75 c.)
- Eggs (2)

How's it done

1. Allow the oven to heat up to 350 degrees. Prepare a baking sheet.
2. Take out a bowl and combine the ingredients. When this is ready, use a tablespoon to scoop out little balls of the dough.
3. Place this into the oven and bake. After 12 minutes, take the bites out and let them cool before serving.

Nutrition
Calories: 159
Fats: 15g
Carbs: 4g
Protein: 2g

Vanilla Pudding

Prep time: 5 minutes
Cooking time: 12 minutes
Servings: 4

What's in it

- Salt
- Vanilla (.5 tsp.)
- Arrowroot flour (1 tsp.)
- Stevia (1.5 tsp.)
- Cream (1 c.)
- Egg yolks (2)

How's it done

1. Combine the egg yolks into a pan and whisk in the vanilla, arrowroot, stevia, and cream. Mix well.
2. Add this to the stove and then reduce the heat when the mixture starts to steam. Stir for ten minutes.
3. After this time, pour the pudding through a mesh sieve into 4 containers. Place in the fridge to store.

Nutrition
Calories: 135
Fats: 13g
Carbs: 2g
Protein: 2g

Poppy Seed Lemon Cupcakes

Prep time: 15 minutes
Cooking time: 30 minutes
Servings: 12

What's in it

- Liquid stevia (1 tsp.)
- Baking powder (2 tsp.)
- Lemon zest (2.5 tsp.)
- Poppy seeds (2 Tbsp.)
- Lemon juice (2.5 Tbsp.)
- Coconut flour (3 oz.)
- Melted butter (4 oz.)
- Greek yogurt (10 oz.)
- Eggs (7)

How's it done

1. Allow the oven to heat up to 375 degrees. Prepare a cupcake tin.
2. Take out bowl and whisk together the stevia, yogurt, and eggs. Add in the butter and set aside.
3. Combine the baking powder and coconut flour and then add to the eggs.
4. Stir the lemon into the batter and the poppy seeds. Pour this into the cupcake tin and place into the oven.
5. After 30 minutes, the cupcakes are done. Allow these to cool before serving.

Nutrition
Calories: 214   Fats: 16g
Carbs: 10g   Protein: 10g

Mint Chocolate Ice Cream

Prep time: 10 minutes
Cooking time:
Servings: 6

What's in it

- Mini chocolate chips (.5 c.)
- Peppermint extract (1 tsp.)
- Vanilla (1 tsp.)
- Stevia (6 tsp.)
- Mint leaves (.25 c.)
- Spinach leaves (.75 c.)
- Coconut cream (1 c.)

How's it done

1. Bring out your blender and add in .25 of the cream in with the mint leaves and spinach leaves. Blend to make creamy.
2. Add the rest of the ingredients into the blender and blend well. Pour into some plastic containers.
3. Keep this in the freezer until the ice cream is set.

Nutrition
Calories: 295
Fat: 31g
Carbs: 5g
Protein: 2.25g

Mango Smoothie

Prep time: 5 minutes
Cooking time: 0 minutes
Servings: 1

What's in it

- Ice cubes (6)
- Sugar (1 Tbsp.)
- Lemon juice (1 Tbsp.)
- Vanilla yogurt (.25 c.)
- Mango juice (.5 c.)
- Mashed avocado (.25 c.)
- Mango cubes (.25 c.)

How's it done

1. Cut the mango into cubes. Cube up the avocado as well.
2. Take out the blender and add in all of the ingredients together. Blend until smooth and then serve.

Nutrition
Calories: 269
Fat: 9g
Carbs: 6g
Protein: 4g

Berry Smoothie

Prep time: 5 minutes
Cooking time: 0 minutes
Servings: 1

What's in it

- Ice (1 c.)
- Water (1 c.)
- Spinach (2 c.)
- Banana (1)
- Raspberries (.25 c.)
- Blueberries (.5 c.)
- Strawberries (.5 c.)

How's it done

1. Chop up the banana, blueberries, raspberries, and strawberries.
2. Bring out the blender and add in the fruits along with the rest of the ingredients.
3. Pour into glasses and serve.

Nutrition
Calories: 218.7
Fat: 13g
Carbs: 20g
Protein: 4.7g

Low Carb Bars

Prep time: 10 minutes
Cooking time: 1 hour
Servings: 16

What's in it

- Dried dates (15)
- Dried fruit (1 c.)
- Nuts (1 c.)

How's it done

1. Allow the oven to heat up to 350 degrees. Roast the nuts until they are browned.
2. Take the seeds out of the dates and then add them, the dried fruit, and nuts to a food processor.
3. Form this into balls and then shape into square shapes on a tray. Place in the fridge for an hour before serving.

Nutrition
Calories: 196
Fat: 9.1g
Carbs: 22g
Protein: 5g

Avocado Tropical Treat

Prep time: 20 minutes
Cooking time: 0 minutes
Servings: 4

What's in it

- Maple syrup (1 drop)
- Natural yogurt, no flavor (.25 c.)
- Sliced kiwi (.5)
- Sliced papaya (.5)
- Sliced banana (.5)
- Diced avocado (.5)

How's it done

1. Take out a bowl and combine the avocado with the fruit.
2. When those are mixed, add in the maple syrup and the yogurt. Mix all of these ingredients together.
3. Add to a blender and puree to a paste form.

Nutrition
Calories: 81
Fat: 6.5g
Carbs: 6.1g
Protein: 1.1g

Keto Lava Cake

Prep time: 5 minutes
Cooking time: 15 minutes
Servings: 1

What's in it

- Vanilla (.5 tsp.)
- Heavy cream (1 Tbsp.)
- Egg (1)
- Erythritol (2 Tbsp.)
- Cocoa powder (2 Tbsp.)
- Salt
- Baking powder (.25 tsp.)

How's it done

1. Allow the oven to heat up to 350 degrees. While that heats up, bring out a bowl and whisk together the erythritol and cocoa powder.
2. In a second bowl, beat the egg. Add this into the erythritol mixture along with the rest of the ingredients.
3. Prepare a few ramekins before adding in the batter. Place into the oven to bake.
4. After 15 minutes, take the cakes out and let them cool down before enjoying.

Nutrition
Calories: 173
Fat: 13g
Carbs: 4g
Protein: 8g

Protein Balls

Prep time: 10 minutes
Cooking time: 30 minutes
Servings: 10

What's in it

- Chocolate protein powder (1 Tbsp.)
- Chia seeds (2 Tbsp.)
- Dark chocolate, chopped (.33 c.)
- Honey (.3 c.)
- Peanut butter (.5 c.)
- Rolled oats (1 c.)

How's it done

1. Mix together the ingredients in a bowl, making sure they are well-combined.
2. Cover these in plastic wrap and let them set in the fridge for half an hour.
3. After this time, take them out and form into balls before serving or storing.

Nutrition
Calories: 188
Fat: 9.9g
Carbs: 21.5g
Protein: 5.8g

Apple Detox

Prep time: 5 minutes
Cooking time:
Servings: 3

What's in it

- Honey (1 tsp.)
- Flax seeds (1 Tbsp.)
- Apple (.5)
- Chopped celery (1 stalk)
- Chopped kale (1.5 c.)
- Ice (.75 c.)
- Almond milk (.66 c.)

How's it done

1. Chop up the apple, celery, and kale. Add these into a blender along with the rest of the ingredients.
2. Blend until these are mixed well, pour into glasses, and serve.

Nutrition
Calories: 50
Fat: 12g
Carbs: 5.7g
Protein: 16g

Raspberry Ice Cream

Prep time: 10 minutes
Cooking time: 10 minutes
Servings: 2

What's in it

- Ice cubes
- Plastic bag (.5 liter)
- Plastic bag (2 liter)
- Rose water (.5 tsp.)
- Vanilla (1 tsp.)
- Raspberries (.3 c.)
- Liquid sweetener (2 Tbsp.)
- Cream (2 c.)
- Salt (.3 c.)

How's it done

1. Take the bigger bag and fill it halfway with cubes. Add the rest of the ingredients to the smaller bag and mix.
2. Add the smaller bag into the bigger one and close it up. Wrap it up in some towels.
3. Shake the bag until the cream turns into an ice cream state. Eat right away.

Nutrition
Calories: 184
Fat: 8.9g
Carbs: 25g
Protein: 2g

Pumpkin Ice Cream

Prep time: 10 minutes
Cooking time: 0 minutes
Servings: 6

What's in it

- Ice cubes (1)
- Pumpkin spice (1.5 tsp.)
- Maple syrup (.3 c.)
- Pumpkin puree (1 c.)
- Frozen bananas (4)

How's it done

1. Take out a blender and add in all of the ingredients, blending until they are mixed well.
2. Pour this into some containers and let it freeze overnight before serving.

Nutrition
Calories: 280
Fat: 20.4g
Carbs: 6.3g
Protein: 4g

Chapter 9: 30-Day Meal Plan to Keep You on Your Goals

Day 1
B: Sausage and Keto Egg Sandwich
L: Chicken Wraps
D: Pumpkin Soup

Day 2
B: Keto Cereal
L: Prosciutto and Brie
D: Super Green Soup

Day 3
B: Ham and Cheese Waffles
L: Keto Cubano
D: Beef Stew

Day 4
B: Eggs and Avocado
L: Monkey Bread
D: Vegetable Dinner

Day 5
B: Bacon Cups
L: Roast Beef Cups
D: Bacon Burgers

Day 6
B: Yogurt Parfait
L: Pork Salad
D: Italian Meatballs

Day 7
B: Cheddar Pancake
L: Chicken Nuggets
D: Beef Welly

Day 8
B: Breakfast Burger
L: Shrimp Salad
D: Salmon Fishcakes

Day 9
B: Scones
L: Mediterranean Tuna
D: Garlic Pork Chops

Day 10
B: Porridge
L: Mac and Cheese
D: Spaghetti

Day 11
B: Scotch Eggs
L: Pork Tenderloin
D: Beef Stew

Day 12
B: Breakfast Tacos
L: Chicken Fingers
D: Vegetable Dinner

Day 13
B: Vanilla Smoothie
L: Ham and Green Bean Salad
D: Shrimp Tuscany

Day 14
B: Blackberry Eggs
L: Cheesy Patties
D: Spaghetti

Day 15
B: Coconut Pancake
L: Mediterranean Tuna
D: Bacon Burgers

Day 16
B: Chocolate Chip Waffles
L: Keto Cubano
D: Pumpkin Soup

Day 17
B: Chocolate and PB Muffins
L: Mac and Cheese
D: Sea Bass

Day 18
B: Butter Coffee
L: Roast Beef Cups
D: Garlic Pork Chop

Day 19
B: Blender Pancakes
L: Feta Cheese Salad
D: Italian Meatballs

Day 20
B: Mocha Chia Pudding:
L: Salmon Potato Salad
D: Eggs and Bacon

Day 21
B: Green Eggs
L: Smoked Salmon
D: Caesar Salad

Day 22
B: Keto Cereal
L: Chicken Wraps
D: Avocado Wedges

Day 23
B: Cheddar Souffle
L: Burgers
D: Beef Chili

Day 24
B: Butter Coffee
L: Blue Bison Burgers
D: Garlic Cod

Day 25
B: Ricotta Pie
L: Blue Cheese Salad
D: Chicken Soup

Day 26
B: Breakfast Tacos
L: Red Salad
D: Shrimp Tuscany

Day 27
B: Scones
L: Black Beans and Rice
D: Ginger Halibut

Day 28
B: Yogurt Parfait
L: Barley Soup
D: Coconut Chicken

Day 29
B: Bacon Cups
L: Smoked Salmon
D: Chicken Skewers

Day 30
B: Ham and Cheese Waffles
L: Red Salad
D: Lamb Chops

Conclusion

Thank you for making it through to the end of this book, let's hope it was informative and able to provide you with all of the tools you need to achieve your goals whatever they may be.

The next step is to get started with your own meal planning adventure! Meal planning is a great way to stay on the ketogenic diet while also ensuring that you save money and time. This guidebook has provided you with the information, as well as the recipes, that you need to make this happen. When you are ready to lose weight on the ketogenic diet and eat right, make sure to check out this guidebook today!

Finally, if you found this book useful in anyway, a review on Amazon is always appreciated!

Recipes Index In Alphabetical Order

Other Books By Elizabeth Wells

Keto Diet For Beginners
Complete Beginner's Guide To Lose Weight Fast And Live Healthier With Ketogenic Cooking

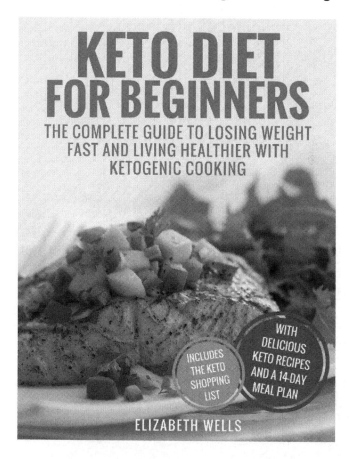

Would you like to lose weight and feel better without only eating salads? Have you already followed countless diets, without actually seeing any results? This one is different, and the results will speak for themselves.

The Ketogenic Diet, or Keto Diet, is a solid dieting

program created back in 1924 by Dr. Russel Wilder and supported by many scientific studies. The Keto Diet is not another diet that promises you everything and delivers you little to nothing! This dieting style lost popularity when some sketchy "lose weight effortlessly" diets came out some years ago, but it is now being acclaimed worldwide again, with famous people following it and new scientific studies being published.

The Keto Diet is based on this principle: your body usually gets energy from the carbs you eat and stores all the excess fats (think about love handles or belly fat). Most diets tell you to stop eating fats to lose weight, however there's a better way to do it.

Some types of fats are healthy and eating them more, while also reducing your intake of carbs, will help you lose weight faster. In fact, if you start eating low carb and high fat your body will use the fats instead of the carbohydrates to produce energy, without actually storing them.

This way, your body will naturally burn fats for you, just by eating the right foods. And the best part is ketogenic foods actually taste really good. Imagine how ketogenic cooking will improve your shape and overall health.

"Once you have been on the ketogenic diet for a few weeks and begun to experience its benefits you will never want to go back to high-carb eating. After all, ketosis is the body's natural state. It's how we were designed to live."

Following this diet is easy when you have the right help. That's why this book will teach you **everything you need to know about the keto diet** to help you lose weight fast and feel better, without being too tricky or complicated. You'll learn exactly what to eat, what to avoid, what recipes to cook, what to store in your pantry to follow the keto diet correctly and start improving your health right now.

Some benefits you'll get by going keto:

- Lose Weight Fast And In A Natural Way
- Feel Better, Both Mentally And Physically
- Eat Healthy Foods That Actually Taste Good
- Have A Healthy, Younger Looking Skin
- Feel Full Of Energy All Day Long
- Lower Your Triglyceride Levels To Prevent Heart Attacks
- Eat Foods That Won't Leave You Hungry All Day
- Improve Your Physical Performance
- Lower Your Cancer Risk
- And Much, Much More

In this book you'll learn:

- What Is The Ketogenic Diet and How It Works
- All The Real Benefits Of The Ketogenic Diet
- A Complete 14-day Keto Meal Plan To Successfully Go Keto
- 20+ Delicious Keto Recipes For Breakfast, Lunch And Dinner
- A List Of Keto Friendly Foods To Store In Your Pantry
- The Complete Keto Shopping List To Fill Your Cart With Healthy Foods
- How To Know If You Shouldn't Follow This Diet
- Simple Tips And Tricks To Stay Keto While

Travelling
- How To Stay On The Keto Diet Through The Holidays
- And Much More

Start improving your health today!

"Keto Diet For Beginners" by Elizabeth Wells is available at Amazon.

Keto Pressure Cooker
101 Delicious Ketogenic Recipes For The Electric Pressure Cooker To Lose Weight Fast And Live Healthier

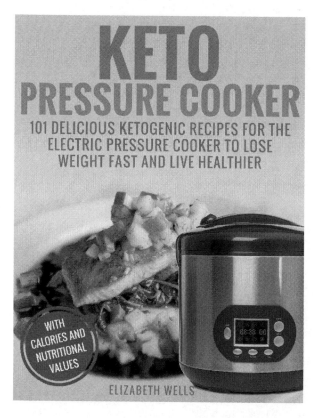

If you love the ketogenic diet and would like to cook dishes using your electric pressure cooker this book is for you. Cooking keto using an electric pressure cooker will help you save time and money without losing the countless benefits of a high fat, low carb diet.

In this cookbook, you'll find 101 mouthwatering ketogenic recipes for every meal time, breakfast, lunch, dinner, sides and desserts. All the recipes include comprehensive instructions and nutritional values, allowing you to know the amount of calories, fats, carbohydrates and proteins contained in each dish.

With the help of these recipes you will easily transition toward a healthier lifestyle.

Some recipes you'll find:
- Korean Steamed Eggs
- Ham And Pepper Fritatta
- Italian Sausage Kale Soup
- Creamy Cauliflower Chowder
- Cream Of Mushroom
- Shredded Chicken
- Green Beans And Bacon
- Prosciutto Wrapped-asparagus
- Coconut Milk Shrimp
- Salmon With Orange Ginger Sauce
- Garlic Cuban Pork
- Garlic And Parmesan Asparagus
- Pumpkin Cheesecake
- Chocolate Mousse
- Coconut Almond Cake
- Chocolate Cheesecake
- And Much More

Enjoy these keto dishes today!

"Keto Pressure Cooker" by Elizabeth Wells is available at Amazon.

Keto Slow Cooker
101 Delicious Ketogenic Recipes For The Slow Cooker To Lose Weight Fast And Live Healthier

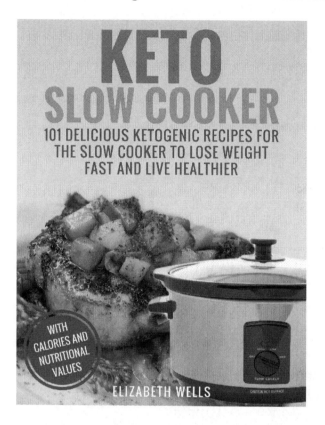

Are you on a ketogenic diet and would love to cook using your slow cooker? Imagine putting a bunch of ingredients in your slow cooker before going to work and coming home to a delicious keto approved meal.

In this cookbook, you'll find 101 delicious ketogenic recipes you can easily cook with your slow cooker. Just follow the simple steps, put all the ingredients in, and let the slow cooker do the rest. You'll discover recipes for chilis, soups, stews, beef meals, poultry and pork dishes, desserts and other tasty treats that will help you save time without losing the countless benefits of a high fat, low carb diet.

All the recipes include step-by-step instructions and nutritional values, allowing you to know the amount of calories, fats, carbohydrates and proteins contained in each dish. And remember, you don't have to spend your entire day in the kitchen to cook healthy dishes.

Some recipes you'll find:
- Chicken Chorizo Soup
- Hare Stew
- BBQ Pulled Beef
- Balsamic Chicken Thighs
- Cuban Ropa Vieja
- Cranberry Pork Roast
- Poached Salmon
- Zucchini Bread
- Chile Verde
- Summertime Veggies
- Jamaican Jerk Roast
- Raspberry Coconut Cake
- Lemon Frosted Cake
- Grain-Free Granola
- And Much More

Enjoy your new recipes today!

"Keto Slow Cooker" by Elizabeth Wells is available at Amazon.

Keto Diet For Beginners
The Step By Step Guide For Beginners To Lose Weight Fast And Live Healthier With The Ketogenic Diet

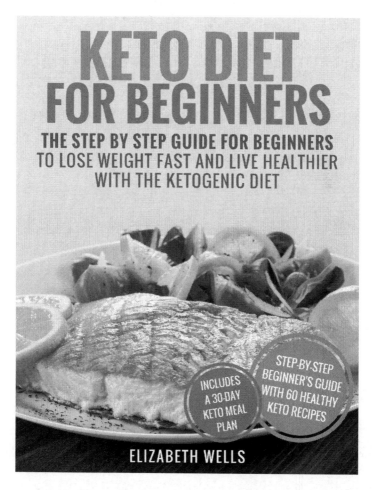

Let's face it, so many people are already in love with this high-fat, low carb diet these days, but there's so much information out there that it can be very overwhelming to figure out how to follow the ketogenic diet without making the most common mistakes.

If you're interested in the keto diet, but don't know where to start, look no further. In this beginner's guide you'll find everything you need to know to start a keto diet and be successful on your dieting journey.

This book will take you step by step through the fundamental principles of the keto diet, will answer all the most common questions and will teach you what foods to eat and what to avoid without being too complicated or overwhelming. After reading this book, you will be well on your way to entering the state known as "ketosis" and jump-starting your new weight loss regimen on the Keto lifestyle.

In this guide you'll find:
- A Step-by-step Process To Start A Keto Diet The Right Way
- History And Fundamental Principles Of The Keto Diet
- How The Ketogenic Diet Works And What You Need To Start Today
- A 30-day Meal Plan Template To Guide You With All The Recipes You Need
- 60 Healthy Ketogenic Recipes For Healthy Breakfast, Lunch, Dinner, Desserts, Snacks And Salads
- A Complete List Of Foods You Should And Shouldn't Eat
- All The Health Benefits You'll Get By Going Keto
- How To Avoid The Common Mistakes All Beginners Make While Starting The Keto Diet
- Ketogenic FAQs: Answers To All The Most Common Questions About The Ketogenic Diet

You will learn all about ketogenic, fasting, weight

loss, and how a low-carb, high-protein diet can change your life mentally, physically, and even emotionally. This book covers its origins as a treatment for epilepsy to all the health problems we face in today's highly processed, fast food world, and how this all contributes to our health. Once you decide to begin a ketogenic diet you will be helping yourself against obesity, diabetes, inflammatory diseases, heart health, curbing dementia, and so much more!

You'll learn how to start the Keto diet successfully with a step-by-step process on how to begin, as well as an extensive list of foods that can and cannot be eaten, so you will be able to know from the start exactly what you should be eating. You'll also find a 30-day meal planning guide along with all the recipes so you can begin planning and hop right away, no need to research for recipes!

Some recipes you'll find in this book:
- Garlic Cedar Plank Salmon
- Prosciutto Wrapped Asparagus
- Tuna Lettuce Wrap With Avocado Yogurt Dressing
- Chicken and Cilantro Salad
- Grilled Salmon with Avocado Bruschetta
- Steak With Balsamic Tomatoes
- California Spicy Crab Stuffed Avocado
- Chicken Pesto Bake
- Zucchini Rolls
- Sausage Stuffed Zucchini with Mozzarella Cheese
- Steak Kebabs with Chimichurri
- Flourless Chocolate Keto Brownies
- Cinnamon Pecan Bars

- Raspberry Lemon Cupcakes
- And Much More

And the best part is, these recipes actually taste good, because remember, being on a diet doesn't have to mean eating flavorless food.

Start the Keto Diet today!

"Keto Diet For Beginners" by Elizabeth Wells is available at Amazon.

Keto Diet
Complete Beginner's Guide To Lose Weight Fast And Live Healthier With Ketogenic Cooking

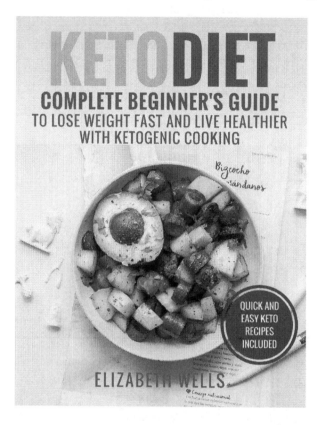

Have you already tried every known diet without seeing any results? Are you willing to lose weight and improve your health but don't want to quit eating some of your loved dishes?

You've come to the right place. The Ketogenic Diet is a popular dieting program that has been around for decades. The Keto Diet is not another fad regime that promises you everything and delivers you little to nothing! This dieting style has been created by Dr. Russell Wilder back in 1924 and is proven and supported by many scientific studies. It lost popularity when some fad "lose weight quick" diets came out some decades ago.

Recently it is being rediscovered and is already acclaimed worldwide. The Keto Diet is well known for being a low carb diet, where the body produces ketones instead of glucose to be used as energy. This will help it burn fats to produce energy without storing them and will drastically reduce the amount of weight you accumulate.

"Eating high fat and low carb offers many health, weight loss, physical and mental performance benefits."

You don't have to quit eating fats to lose weight. You'll still be able to enjoy food that actually tastes good and makes you happy.

In this book you'll learn how the Keto Diet works and how you can start improving your health right now by cooking delicious dishes.

These are some of the benefits you'll get:

- Lose weight naturally and easily
- Feel well, both mentally and physically
- Keep your skin younger looking
- Eat healthy foods you actually like
- Satisfy your appetite without remaining hungry all day
- Achieve a lower blood pressure
- Prevent heart attacks by lowering your triglyceride levels
- Increase your energy and improve your physical performance
- Lower your cancer risk

- And much more

Following this diet without any help can be complex, especially if you're a beginner. That's why this book aims to teach you everything you need to know to improve your eating habits and your life, without being too tricky or complicated.

In this book you'll learn:

- What is the Ketogenic Diet
- What You Should Eat (And What You Shouldn't)
- 43 Recommended Foods (with calories, grams of carbs, proteins and fats contained)
- How To Follow The Keto Diet Correctly (Most People Get This Wrong)
- 3 Signs That You've Reached Ketosis
- The Benefits Of Going Keto
- 50 Quick And Easy To Cook Keto Recipes
- And much more

What are you waiting for? Start eating healthier today!

"Keto Diet" by Elizabeth Wells is available at Amazon.

Ketogenic Diet Guide For Beginners:

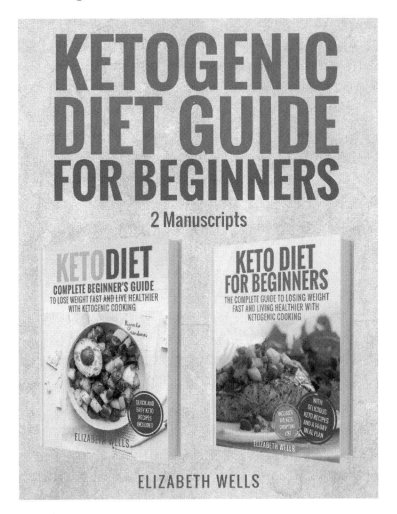

"Ketogenic Diet Guide For Beginners" by Elizabeth Wells is available at Amazon.

Made in the USA
Lexington, KY
02 June 2018